Medical Writing: a Prescription for Clarity

This is the third edition of a book that discusses style but is mostly about communication. Effective communication is the ultimate, but often daunting, purpose of any piece of medical research. This very helpful book provides practical information enabling first drafts to be turned into concise unambiguous text, without loss of individuality. Written by a consultant anaesthetist and an experienced medical editior, it is sympathetic to the problems and needs of medical writers. Like the preceding two editions, this expanded third edition deals with the basic craft of writing for publication, from spelling and grammar to choosing the best word or phrase.

Whether you are writing a simple clinical report or thesis, want to supervise others or just want to develop greater skill in effective writing, this book is the ideal guide and reference. Clear, simple and precise, and illustrated with apt cartoons, this is an invaluable handbook.

From Reviews of previous editions.

'engagingly written' *BMJ.*

'This book is packed with little gems. It provides not only excellent advice but highly enjoyable bedtime reading. Indeed, it is one of the most enjoyable texts I have read in recent times' *British Journal of Anaesthesia.*

'Anyone who aspires to medical or scientific authorship should read this book' *Journal of the Institution of Health Education.*

DR NEVILLE GOODMAN is currently Consultant Anaesthetist at Southmead Hospital, Bristol.

DR MARTIN EDWARDS, previously Senior Research Fellow at the Royal College of Surgeons of England, is currently a freelance medical editor.

DR ANDY BLACK, now retired, was Senior Lecturer in Anaesthesia at Bristol University.

Medical Writing

A Prescription for Clarity

THIRD EDITION

DR NEVILLE W. GOODMAN

Consultant Anaesthetist, Southmead Hospital, Bristol

DR MARTIN B. EDWARDS

Freelance Medical Editor (formerly Senior Research Fellow, Royal College of Surgeons of England)

and with cartoons by

DR ANDY BLACK

Retired Senior Lecturer in Anaesthesia, Bristol University

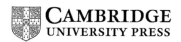

CAMBRIDGE
UNIVERSITY PRESS

CAMBRIDGE UNIVERSITY PRESS
Cambridge, New York, Melbourne, Madrid, Cape Town, Singapore, São Paulo

Cambridge University Press
The Edinburgh Building, Cambridge CB2 2RU, UK

Published in the United States of America by Cambridge University Press, New York

www.cambridge.org
Information on this title: www.cambridge.org/9780521858571

First published 1991
Second edition 1997
Third edition 2006

Printed in the United Kingdom at the University Press, Cambridge

A catalogue record for this book is available from the British Library

ISBN-13 978-0-521-85857-1 paperback
ISBN-10 0-521-85857-7 paperback

This third edition is rededicated to the memory of

Bob Torrance

and

Brian Phythian

who between them are largely responsible for everything in it.

It is also, sadly, dedicated to the memory of my co-author Martin, who died during its production. Martin and I shared views on English, and never once had a disagreement about anything while preparing all three editions. Although the book was my idea, his talent for sanding down my sharp edges is the reason that the first edition was published, and that another two have followed. Thanks to everything. [NWG]

We have frequent occasion to observe this tendency to neologism, and the avidity with which [writers] cover a certain crudity of reasoning and obscurity of thought, or endeavour to give weight to a shallow theory, by the selection of the very longest and most technical words which the medical vocabulary will supply. This is an error to be deplored and reprobated.

The *Lancet* 30 Sept 1885: quoted in the column 'From The Lancet' *Lancet* 1990; 336: 224.

It is remarkably easy not to say what you mean.

Appleton, D. R. Cross words. *Br. Med. J.* 1994; 309: 1737–8.

The first (and rarest) quality is brevity: short words, short sentences. Why is it that intelligent people (among whom I include doctors) become imbued with verbosity the moment they put pen to paper?

Paton, A. In *How to Do It: 1.* London: BMJ Publishing Group, 1985, pp. 207–11.

The more precisely we speak, the more effectively we are able to communicate our meaning to others. The English language has rules of grammar and individual words have definitions to facilitate effective communication.

Halperin, E. C. The right verb. *Int. J. Radiation Oncol. Biol. Phys.* 1987; 13: 143.

People who write obscurely are either unskilled in writing or up to some mischief.

Medawar, P. *The Threat and the Glory*, ed. Pyke D. Oxford: Oxford University Press, 1990, p. xv.

Contents

Preface to the first edition

Doctors, nurses, paramedical workers and medical scientists need to communicate their ideas effectively. Writers in the field of medicine tend to use unfamiliar words in tortuous constructions, particularly when writing reports for submission to learned journals. Research can often be judged only by its final written report. A meticulous study can be let down by poor writing, which may lead a reviewer to wonder if lack of attention to detail in the writing indicates lack of attention to detail in the research. Certain usually superfluous words and phrases occur again and again in medical papers. Once able to recognize these, writers should be able to delete them or to find more appropriate constructions, guided by the suggestions made in this book.

Most of the examples are quotations from medical books and journals, though some, particularly those from more specialized texts, have been modified.

Words or phrases whose use in medical writing is discussed specifically in the text are in capitals:

   a where they occur as the 'heading' to a main entry, i.e. where the discussion takes place;

   b in cross-references to main entries, for example '(see REGIME)';

   c in the index.

Superscript numbers in the text refer to articles and books listed sequentially in the reference list at the end of the book. There is also a list of the standard texts to which we refer frequently, and these texts are identified by author's name or by an obvious shorthand: for instance, Greenbaum and Whitcut are the latest revisers of Sir Ernest Gowers' *The Complete Plain Words*, and this is referred to as *Gowers*. *COD* is the *Concise Oxford Dictionary*.

Preface to the third edition

For the second edition, we included more examples and exercises, and a new chapter on that much abused diagram, the graph. For the third, there are new examples and fresh exercises. There are a number of new entries for words that we overlooked or have since and inadvisably become more prevalent. In the 15 years since the first edition, we have not detected any great change in the attitudes of medical writers to the way they write. For this reason, the introductory chapters, which attempt to explain the reasons for poor medical writing, remain much as they were in the previous two editions.

Some attitudes to higher education may make the book even more necessary in the future. Frank Furedi[1] quotes a professor of education who believes essay writing is elitist and that it is, therefore, unfair to ask university students to write them. Educationalists are having an increasing influence in undergraduate and postgraduate medical education in the United Kingdom; there is also the perceived preference of medical schools for 'privileged' students, which politicians want to prevent. These influences may make it even more difficult for future doctors to express themselves well on paper.

Frontline journals are receiving more papers now from authors whose first language is not English. We did not mention these EFL (English as a foreign language) authors in earlier editions, and it is not easy to cater for the different grammars that these authors carry mistakenly into their English. However, many of the faults in medical English are stereotyped and common: much of the effort of correcting them is in pattern recognition. Such authors should profit from reading this book rather than dipping into it. They will have picked up the bad habits of writing largely from reading the bad writing of others, rather than for the reasons given in our introductory chapters. They can, therefore, feel somewhat aggrieved to have been so corrupted, but we hope to uncorrupt them within our pages.

Some of our previously recommended texts are in new editions, but some are now out of print. Since our first edition appeared, other new books have also appeared, but these are listed only if they came to our attention for some reason; we do not intend to give a comprehensive list of books on writing English.

Acknowledgements

Many people have helped with this book, wittingly or unwittingly. Most of the examples are quotations from medical books and journals and we thank the writers for them; while they may recognize their own words, we hope others will be unable to make an attribution.

Earlier versions of the first edition were seen by a number of assessors, usually reviewers reporting to publishers. Many of their comments were added to the text and again they may be recognized. Because the reviewers were anonymous, we can do no more than give a general thanks.

PART I

Problem: the illness

1
Introduction

This book is about words: about the ways in which words are used by doctors, medical scientists and others who write on medical matters. These ways are mostly no different from the ways that words are used and misused in many other subjects. But, in our opinion, too many of the producers and consumers of academic medical English are tolerant of writing that is clumsy, inaccurate, obscure or just downright bad. The first section of this book examines the roots of that tolerance; the remainder and larger part deals with the nuts and bolts of writing, taking its numerous examples from the field of medicine.

Our approach is to encourage good writing by examining bad writing, because it is often easier to say what is bad about a piece of writing than what is good. This sentiment is shared by Bernard Dixon, who compiled a collection of unarguably well-written scientific articles from past and present.[2] In his preface, he says of bad writing, 'We can learn important lessons by inspecting such specimens, just as pathologists learn from even the most unattractive objects and tissues that arrive in their laboratories.' This book contains collections of these specimens and a record of their dissections.

What constitutes good or bad writing is not easy to define. How to distinguish between good and bad without sounding didactic or arrogant is a challenge. In applying judgemental words – 'good', 'bad', 'clumsy', 'pompous' and others – to examples of writing, we accept that we are making value judgements. But we are actually more concerned with *valid* judgements and we leave it to readers to test the validity of our criticisms against their own values. Certainly no plea is made here that words have inviolable meanings and that we should all go back pedantically to their etymological roots to define meanings for evermore. For example, the original meaning of the word *decimate* was *to put to death one in ten*, but *decimate* has now come to mean *to destroy a large proportion* and the original meaning has been lost.

If any plea is entered it is on behalf of clear, simple, unambiguous writing. That whatever word is used should be, as far as possible, the correct word, chosen for its precise meaning that everyone understands. Words that are changing their meanings may mean different things to different people, and it is for this reason – not because they appreciate the finer points of etymology – that good writers will avoid them.

If there is a simple maxim for good medical writing, it is that almost always the better word is shorter and the better construction has fewer words.

The intent of this book is, then, largely practical. Some of the technical exercises involve that most practical of modern writing tools, the word processor. At the simplest level, the aim of the prescriptive lists in the book is to help writers to realize that it is easy to make a start at improvement. The lists are of suggested better words and better constructions, where better means clearer and more precise. If writers used the lists in this simple way, their writing would surely improve, but there is a more important reason for the book: to show that there is no difference between clear, precise thinking and clear, precise writing.

That much of medical writing is bad does not mean that the writers, particularly those with little experience, should bear all the blame. Bad writing is contagious if the reader has not received an adequately immunizing dose of good. The practical exercises in this book are intended to begin the process of acquiring resistance. Readers queuing for their first shot of vaccine but at this stage less concerned with the immunopathology of writing may choose to move directly to the next section – with both sleeves rolled up. Later, sustained by high titres of antijargon, we hope they will return to the more philosophical considerations of the next chapter.

2

The malaise of medical manuscripts

We think in words. We form our ideas in words. If doctors write descriptions of clinical trials that confuse readers assumed to be of equal knowledge and understanding, then that is the responsibility of the writers not the readers, who might justifiably wonder whether the conduct of the clinical trials had been similarly confused. (The difference between 're-sponsibility' and 'fault' serves a purpose here. We have already indicated that writers should not necessarily be blamed for their bad habits.)

Medicine is a practical subject so here is an example of confused writing, taken from a clinical report. The investigators were relating the rate of infusion of a drug to its concentration in the blood. They wrote,

> The infusion rate was then increased and blood was taken 4, 8, 12, and 20 minutes *after* [our italics] the new target concentration had been achieved.

The meaning of this sentence is clear: they wanted there to be a higher concentration of drug, which would have a greater effect, and blood was taken to ascertain what happened after the new, desired concentration had been reached. This is a reasonable thing to want to know; after all, if the concentration varied, then the effect could be unpredictable.

The meaning is absolutely clear; but the trouble is that it is not what the investigators meant. They were interested in how quickly the concentration reached its new steady state after the rate of infusion had been increased; they took blood 4, 8, 12 and 20 minutes after taking the action that sought to produce a new target concentration, that is, after altering the rate of infusion. To do the experiment as described they would have needed to know the concentration at the time of sampling. This may be possible eventually, using quantitative methods *in vivo*, but these investigators did not know the concentration of the drug in the blood until *after analysis* some days later. What they should have written is, *The infusion rate was then increased and blood was taken 4, 8, 12, and 20 minutes later*, or (although it is implicit and not strictly necessary) . . . *after the new target concentration had been set.*

Science depends on clear thinking and accurate reporting. These investigators described the defining of a future event as the achievement of that event – they described aiming at the target as hitting the target. Is it unfair to wonder if their scientific method might have been similarly imprecise?

Sadly, an editorialist at the *British Medical Journal* was not being ironic when writing a comment on a doctor struck off the medical register for faking ethics committee approval for a research project, 'The forgeries were described as "hopelessly inept", containing grammatical errors and couched in language that was difficult to understand'. If the doctor had managed to do the research, such skill would have made the forged research pretty well undetectable.

The writer at bay

The first response of writers when their writing is criticized is likely to be one of indignation. This is not surprising. First, most people assume they can express themselves in their mother tongue. (It is unfair to be over-critical when writers are not writing in their first language.) Second, however unimportant the question, slovenly the method and inappropriate the conclusions may appear to the reader, a paper being prepared for a medical journal is the report of work that has taken time and effort. It is not easy to tell parents that their child is stupid.

Whatever the particular criticism, whether of incorrect use of a single word or of impenetrable paragraphs of 'pseudo-scientific' prose, there are five defences that authors commonly proffer.

- Everyday language is inappropriate and not precise enough to describe the results of a medical study.
- Long words are more scientific.
- Their writing style follows the convention for writing medical papers.
- However writers write, editors will alter the writing to suit themselves.
- Everyone has their own style, and to use this style is better than conforming to a supposedly correct set of rules.

The first two are the defences most often used by aggrieved writers; the others are less common but no less pernicious. All five are inadequate but, for our purposes, illustrative.

Everyday language

There is some justification in the claim that everyday language is inappropriate, because sometimes it is. Colloquial expressions such as *mum* for *mother*, *kid* for *child*, and *swig* for *drink* would be out of place in formal writing, but that does not mean that all simple words are similarly condemned. There is no good reason for choosing *maternal parent, paediatric patient* and *liquid imbibition*: or for claiming that these longer substitutions are more precise. There is no more precise way of expressing the idea of a female parent than the word *mother*. To prefer *liquid imbibition* to *drink* (-ing) is a pompous inflation not often encountered. The *paediatric patient* is now a common visitor to medical texts and more problematic. Is he or she a child or an adolescent; is there a global standard age range for the paediatric category? (See p. 152.) It may be necessary to be more precise and use more words when a shorthand form, however familiar, is also ambiguous.

Precise, therefore, does not always mean *short*, although the more precise word of a pair is commonly the shorter one. *Precise* means *accurately expressed*. Something that is precise will be clear and unambiguous, which is what is needed in scientific or medical writing. We tend to avoid long words and complicated constructions in everyday speech with colleagues and patients, largely because these words and constructions are imprecise, inefficient and difficult to understand, and we should do the same in our writing. It is also nonsense, and arrogant, to claim that the words we use in medical articles and books should be different from everyday usage in case patients try to read them; that is going back to the Middle Ages, when to know the name of something was to have power over it.

There is a story, often quoted, about a child who was asked to describe a cow and wrote:

> A cow is an animal with four legs, and horns on its head. Grass goes in at the head end and manure comes out at the tail end.

Somewhere between primary school and our postgraduate medical examinations something goes sadly wrong, because by then we may be capable of writing:

Follow-up clinics should be subjected to critical analysis in terms of the efficiency and effectiveness of the care provided.

instead of *We need to assess the efficiency and effectiveness of follow-up clinics*, or *We need to know whether follow-up clinics are efficient and effective* or, what we really think, which is, 'Are follow-up clinics worthwhile?'

Long words and scientific conventions

Are longer words more scientific, a reason commonly given for their use? *Roget's Thesaurus*, in one of its lists of words with similar and allied meanings, has *accurate, meticulous, delicate, undeviating* and *sensitive* in the same section as *scientific*, but it does not have synonyms such as *complicated, complex, contorted,* or *long winded.* The *COD* defines *scientific* as 'according to rules laid down in exact science for performing observations and testing soundness of conclusions, systematic, accurate', and *science* is described as 'systematic and formulated knowledge'.

Science can be very complicated, but there is nothing in its definition that implies it must be, or that requires descriptions of science to be written in any sort of special language that only scientists understand. (We consider the rhetorical aspects of scientific writing later (pp. 10 and 26).) The detail and implications of Einstein's theory of relativity may be beyond the understanding of many of us, but it can be described in simple language, which is what Einstein himself used in his own writing.

Complex language makes understanding even more difficult. There have been many developments in physics since Einstein, and there will be few clinicians who can grasp the intricacies of, say, the more recent theory of superstrings. This requires an understanding of a number of dimensions beyond the familiar three, and attempts to explain, in the same physical terms, time, mass, gravity and other phenomena. Complex the theory may be, but when an editorial appeared about it in the *Lancet*[3] the writing was a model of clarity:

Since 1984, there has been an explosion of enthusiasm for superstring theory, motivated by indications that this theory will not only lead to a consistent understanding of quantum gravity but also necessarily unify all the fundamental particles and the physical forces. The basic principle is that the fundamental particles (e.g., the electron, the quarks, and other particles) are extended, string-like, objects rather

> than the structureless point-like objects that appear in all previous quantum theories (e.g., those based on Maxwell's electromagnetism or Einstein's gravity). . .
>
> . . .For general reasons, in a complete quantum theory that includes gravity along with the other forces, [the] familiar notion of space-time must be altered. . .[and]. . .can no longer be considered as a smooth collection of points but is continuously fluctuating in a manner that depends on the forces exerted by the particles that move through it.

The theory is mind-boggling; the idea of space–time fluctuation is certainly beyond easy comprehension. But the expression of these ideas could not be more clear, and it can be grasped readily at first reading. The clarity gives the subject immediacy and makes it interesting. It leaves the reader curious to know more. There is no reason at all why a medical paper should not read like a *Lancet* editorial.

Compare that passage with this next extract, which is about the control of breathing. All workers in medicine will have some idea of the physiology of breathing and so should have a grasp of the terminology (which we may lack in subatomic physics).

> A speculative proposal that the physiological explication of the control of pulmonary ventilation in the mammal is made coherent and consistent with most physiological observation if the control conceptualization is formulated around the notion that air flow is the real part of an analytic time varying signal. The instantaneous amplitude and phase of the signal correspond to depth and rate of breathing.

The writer has used the word *coherent*, which means, among other things, *easily followed*. Ironic, then, that the expression of these ideas, compared with the nominally more difficult ones from particle physics, could not be more opaque, and the ideas are impossible to grasp at first reading. The opacity makes the reader eager to skip the rest of the article. In fact, the extraordinarily contorted first sentence can be summed up quite simply:

> *All observations relating to the control of breathing in the mammal can be explained in terms of the instantaneous air flow.*

The original, though nearly impossible to understand, would probably be said by many to be more scientific.

There is a circular argument here: it is science that is reported in journals; journals contain heavy, polysyllabic, impressive-sounding prose;

therefore, this style of writing is scientific. The inevitable conclusion is that this style must be used when writing medical and scientific papers.

Is scientific style just a matter of convention? Is it essential to follow that convention in order to communicate effectively? Clearly there are structures that contribute to making scientific communications 'universally' intelligible. An obvious example, above the level of sentences and their order, is the sequence of sections (Introduction, Materials and Methods, and so on) common to papers in many journals. However, down in the dirt among the words and punctuation there are other, less obvious but insidious, structures that have the guise of conventions but which all too easily produce stylistic obscurity. And these are certainly self-perpetuating. If papers in the journals are written badly, aspiring authors are likely to copy the style and write badly themselves. A convention that makes writing less clear cannot make for good science and, therefore, has no use. A convention that has no use should be abandoned.

Certain conventions in scientific writing endure for good reasons. For example, there is little place for style that imparts mood and emotion to the words; we are reporting facts, and stating opinions based on them and their relation to other facts. But even this requirement for 'scientific objectivity' may yield to literary analysis by detached observers. John Durant[4] quotes from Alan Gross's *The Rhetoric of Science*: 'The objectivity of scientific prose is a carefully crafted rhetorical invention, a nonrational appeal to the authority of reason.' This is too large a subject to debate further here (see p. 20), but we suggest that clear and simple words can expose irrationality as powerfully as they can endorse objectivity. We may need to remember too that the Internet can give the so-called lay public far greater access than before to scientific pronouncements. These readers in cyberspace may prove to be harsh and demanding critics, with well-developed sensitivity to the 'authority of reason' and every justification for scepticism about scientism rather than science. The medical writer needs to think about this new audience.

Less controversially, there is more room for personal style in reviews and books. For reviewing, the style used for bare scientific reporting removes the whole purpose, which is to be critical. As Sam Shuster[5] wrote in a book review, 'In each of the three books mediocrity of approach showed itself in the fear of personal involvement and commitment and in the curious and almost reverential equality accorded to all published work.'

Shuster's comment is pertinent to our case. There is a tendency to revere the printed word and with it its conventions, whether they serve a useful function or not. We write the way we do because of what we read; but we also write in a way we think is expected. This harks back to the idea (Chapter 1) that bad writing is contagious. Part of the protection against this would be to widen our reading. Max Perutz[6], Peter Medawar[7] and Richard Feynman[8] all won Nobel prizes for scientific discoveries. They did not write a special kind of scientific prose; they wrote clear, simple English. Perhaps they should be among our models. They wrote clear, simple English to express clear, simple thoughts, even though the subjects they researched were at times complex and perplexing. They did not think of 'speculative proposals' and 'physiological explications'.

Perutz quotes Medawar in saying that good writing is almost always shorter than bad. Feynman tells a story in his autobiography[8] of a conversation he had with a stenotypist at a conference of social scientists. He asked Feynman about his profession and was surprised when Feynman told him he was a professor.

> 'Of what?'
> 'Of physics – science.'
> 'Oh, that must be the reason,' he said.
> 'Reason for what?'
> He said, 'You see, I'm a stenotypist, and I type everything that is said here. Now, when the other fellas talk, I type what they say, but I don't understand what they're saying. But every time you get up to ask a question or to say something, I understand exactly what you mean – what the question is, and what you're saying – so I thought you *can't* be a professor!'

Better to emulate the professor of physics than these particular social scientists.

The interfering editor

It is all very well to suggest that writers aim at simplicity and, with a brave pen or keystroke, begin to change medical writing for the better. But what if those to whom they submit their work make no great distinction between good and bad writing, and are themselves slaves to conventions? In other words: who is better placed to effect change, the writer or the editor and publisher? Here are chicken and egg, and the question is clearly rhetorical, but worth asking none the less. Good writers presumably exercise better quality control over their work than bad, but there are very few writers in any field who have not benefited from the attention of an editor, even if only to reinforce their own certainty that they are getting it right without outside interference. And publishers through their editors can deploy the ultimate sanctions – to accept or not, to alter or not, to publish *and* be damned.

Here we ought to make some distinction between the title of editor and the function of editing. Editors of journals have ultimate power in accepting or rejecting submitted papers but they do not necessarily edit them in the sense of making them clearer and shorter. Arguably that editorial function is the province of editorial assistants, subeditors, copy-editors and the like. Although writers may complain when their writing is altered by 'editors', such changes – the process of subediting – are usually an improvement. It is rare for subeditors to rewrite papers radically. In our experience, it is also rare for them to make a paper worse by deliberately inserting the more turgid of 'scientific conventions' if the writer has avoided them. Usually they correct serious grammatical errors and alter particular phrases to conform to the 'house style' of the journal (which will include the representation of numbers and units, illustrations and tables, and references). Any alterations usually make the text simpler and more precise than the original.

Editors and their panels of accepting editors are sometimes a different kettle of fish. We assume they do not prefer pseudo-scientific writing, but many are partly responsible for it because they appear to take no action to change it. Gregory[9] believes that editors should be writers not scientists, and that badly written work should be rejected, whatever its scientific standard. His is clearly not a widely accepted view: the problem with many journals is that they seem not to be subedited at all. The writing in some of the specialized journals is particularly bad, and it is difficult to avoid thinking that the editors are concerned only with filling the pages. As O'Donnell[10] put it, 'some journals propagate language that not only obstructs understanding but allows authors to indulge in sloppy thinking'. We agree with Gregory: editors of medical and scientific journals should have a feel for language, and themselves be able to write well. Being a good clinician, a well-known specialist, having many published papers, or wanting to add an editorship to the curriculum vitae is not enough.

Editors may be too busy to do the subediting themselves, but there is a strong argument that they must be capable of it. If, as many do, they use the help of colleagues, then those colleagues should also be able to write effectively. Some editors use professional but non-medical subeditors, whose unfamiliarity with the detail of the subject can sometimes lead to changes in meaning. This is usually noticed when the proof of the script arrives, and writers should then inform the editor. If the writer is not feeling too churlish, they may incline to agree that their paper has been improved, even if a scientific detail or two has been temporarily misplaced.

The referees to whom editors send manuscripts for assessment must also bear some responsibility for poor writing. Referees should criticize bad writing. Editors should send papers back to authors for rewriting, even papers that have been judged scientifically sound. This requires that the referees and editors are able to recognize bad writing. They should also have a feel for the distinction between 'bad' writing, which is a matter of sometimes subjective judgement, and writing whose difficulties reflect that English is not the writer's first language. Editing second-language texts for clarity is demanding work, but important if the international project in medical communication is to flourish.

It would be laughably naive not to acknowledge that active editing is time consuming and therefore expensive (even when the time devoted is not actually paid for by the publisher). In fact the lack of 'cost-effectiveness' in subediting (and the lack of subeditors) is often given as the reason for not doing it at all or well. Publishers must take responsibility for this state of affairs when they stray from their traditional role of selecting, making and marketing a product of excellence. The various kinds of medical text may have different levels of profitability. Some may be viable only within the broader context of the commercial success of the whole publishing enterprise. This is not an argument for producing more and worse rather than better but possibly less. The extent to which some of the output in medical communication is worth publishing in the first place is surely bound up with the quality of the writing and editing, though not wholly dependent upon it.

Personal style

There remains one from the list of five defences of impenetrable prose: that it is better to write with a personal style than to conform to a set of rules. Underlying this is the idea that obeying rules leads to dull uniformity. Authors who make this claim almost always have no idea of what the rules are but, more importantly, often no one will have given them any advice. They refer to no authority when asked why they have used a particular word or construction because they know of no authority; the stock answer is that it means the same anyway.

What they are doing, perhaps unknowingly, is obeying a set of unwritten rules: the conventions (again) of pseudo-scientific writing. Too often, these conventions demand that the simple statement, for example, *Cocaine causes addiction*, is replaced by the circumlocutory – *It has been shown that cocaine causes addiction*. There is no need for the extra words: we cannot know if cocaine causes addiction unless someone has shown it. It is just a matter of style, but does anyone think the longer sentence is the better style? We hope not, because verbose style can change meaning. When writers write *It has been shown that cocaine is associated with addiction*, they may mean *Cocaine causes addiction* (or, better, *Cocaine is addictive*) but it is important to realize that association is not causation. Petty theft is also associated with addiction, as is AIDS. However, petty theft does not cause addiction; it is the addiction that drives the theft. Cocaine and AIDS are both associated with addiction, but associations between cocaine and AIDS are likely to be indirect because cocaine addicts do not use the drug intravenously. Confusing association and causation is a common error in medical writing (see p. 184).

Good writers of medical English still manage to write with style, but they write on a base of good English. Enthusiastic writers will inevitably instil something personal into their writing, even when what is written is a formal, academic communication. Robert Barrass,[11] wrote: 'There is no one correct way to write, since the way each person puts words together to convey meaning reflects their personality and their feeling for words.'

In most discussions about words, writers at bay tend to turn on their challengers with the riposte: 'Why is your word any better? They mean the same, and you knew what I meant.' The answer is: because the writing is the only representation of the science that the readers will see; writing and science cannot be separated. Investigators design protocols for studies and have to be able to reply to criticism of the design. They can be criticized for inaccurate measurements; they must be able to justify their statistical methods. Criticisms and challenges of these things are expected, yet criticisms of the writing are too often seen as distracting from the science. When writers write in a particular way, when they have chosen certain words to describe their studies, the words and the writing are their responsibility as much as the protocol, the measurements and the statistics. Readers have a right to accurate, clear descriptions without having constantly to look back to previous sentences, or to interpret the meaning of words from their contexts. Excessive fussing about details of wording is commonly dismissed, particularly at medical meetings, as nit picking, yet science depends on meticulous attention to detail.

Investigators will often answer a query about their study by referring to other work or to textbooks, or by producing a slide they had in reserve. Yet rarely do they attempt to justify the use of an incorrect word, other than by bluster. It is obvious that the writing has been seen as unimportant: just the tedious business of getting it down on paper. Robert Barrass[11] wrote, 'Some scientists do not write as well as they should because they do not think of writing as part of science.' Sadly, many doctors and medical scientists seem unaware that any advice about writing is available, yet alone easy to obtain.

This ignorance is obvious from a common phrase in pseudo-scientific writing: *prior to* instead of *before*. *Prior to* appears in most books on English usage and is universally condemned (unless used to convey *more* than just a *temporal* sense of preceding), which must mean that medical writers who use *prior to* have not read any books on English usage. While it requires practice to be able to rewrite 'The frequency of acute carbon monoxide intoxication at home remains high' as the simpler and more direct *Acute poisoning by carbon monoxide in the home is still common*, avoiding *prior to* is easy.

Yes, *prior to* means *before*. It is listed in the *COD*. By all means write *One injection of a depot insulin prior to breakfast may provide reasonable control* if you tell your children to go and wash their hands prior to dinner, but we prefer to follow the advice of authorities on English usage and to write *before*.

In fact, the example of *prior to* is a plank in a wider argument. The phrase is, perhaps, encountered more often in spoken and written American rather than UK English. But there are signs that it is becoming more common in UK English (especially in the sciences), possibly by attraction or imitation. (We fear that people are tending more and more to say *prior to* instead of *before* in everyday speech, and that this tendency has accelerated since the first edition.) This might be an example of language in dynamic change; it might also be a small indicator that American English will, as widely predicted, become the dominant form of English in scientific communication, particularly for those whose first language is not English. No value judgement is intended by these comments: if in some sense *prior to* is not good English, its inadequacies are not directly from being used rather more in American English. The best of that language brings a conciseness and vigour to scientific writing, just as it does to fiction. No, the spread of *prior to* as an example of infection in bad writing is more to do with its associations than its origins. *Prior to* has become one of the signals of turgid bureaucratic prose, of what the cynical may regard as deliberate attempts to confuse and obscure by euphemism, of Pentagonese and Whitehall-speak (see below and Lutz[12]).

Even those who disagree with this conclusion might concede that *prior to* is now common in the written and spoken news media on this side of the Atlantic. To those who work closely with words, there are signs that, in recent scientific and medical writing, the *most important sources* of vocabulary and grammar are limited to those media, and to other pieces of scientific writing. With this sort of restriction in literary experience, it should be no surprise that the infection of bad writing is rife.

The honest writer

Medical and scientific reporting must be honest, which is another and formidable reason why words should be chosen and used with care. Politicians make meaningless statements such as, 'The Iranian government in all its dimensions is helping with the hostage crisis', and estate agents describe houses as 'deceptively spacious'. The *Independent* newspaper of 15 September 1990 quoted a managing director as saying of a scheme for loans to students, 'This is not lending. This is giving money as part of an educational expansion programme. The fact that the student has to pay the money back is the only resemblance to a loan.' Which makes a mortgage not a loan but a 'housing expansion project'.

We may choose to ascribe particular and not necessarily benign motives to people who say and write these things; there is no place for similar motives in research. Facts must be reported for what they are, which means they must be reported with all their loose ends. It is easy to ignore observations because they do not fit preconceived ideas, or because they are awkward outliers that spoil the conclusion. But the observations are the reason for the report. Richard Feynman[8] wrote:

> It's a kind of scientific integrity, a principle of scientific thought that corresponds to a kind of utter honesty – a kind of leaning over backwards. For example, if you're doing an experiment, you should report everything that you think might make it invalid – not only what you think is right about it. . . . In summary, the idea is to try to give all of the information to help others to judge the value of your contribution; not just the information that leads to judgement in one particular direction or another.

It follows from this that not only must all the information be given but it must also be given clearly and simply and without attempts to influence readers. To quote Feynman again, 'The first principle is that you must not fool yourself – and you are the easiest person to fool.'

There are many ways that scientific and medical writers try to fool themselves. A common one is to present numerical observations in a favourable light, perhaps by reporting the mean of a measured variable without giving its variability. This is omitting 'information to help others to judge the value of your contribution'. As with statistics, so with language: everything that is written must be chosen precisely and not left to be puzzled over by the readers. Newspapers carry advertisements for financial loans in which interest payments are quoted commonly as 'only £50 per month for 120 months'. This is £600 per year for 10 years; it is quoted intentionally as months because 120 months seem less than 10 years: without doing the mental arithmetic, how long is 100000 seconds? Medical scientists presenting their results should not risk being accused of having the motives of moneylenders or the guile of politicians, both being part of the strategy of selling and designed to cause confusion – they have no part in the communication of facts. As the Conservative politician the late Alan Clark wrote of the arms to Iraq affair in the 1990s, 'The trouble is that the "ordinary meaning of words" and natural common sense and other familiar devices which we employ in ordinary [dealings between people], have deliberately been avoided. . .'.

Confused thinking and confused writing may produce not just confused readers but confused medical practice.[13] The implications of clinical research, and the inferences we make from it, alter treatments and affect patients. The clearer the language, the less likely that errors of logic will be made in drawing conclusions from studies. Perhaps this is another good reason for remembering that medical writing now reaches a wider, 'lay' audience that is increasingly seeking information to inform and empower its choices as equal participants in prevention and treatment.

Researchers want to discover things, and those who give practical or financial support to research want a return for their support. These are strong forces towards a piece of research having to provide an answer: more than that, an answer that matters. It is these forces that are responsible for some of the errors of logic in the interpretation of medical research. The simplest errors of interpretation come from the misuse of statistics, but there are other errors of logic that are not so simple, that depend on thoughts and words rather than figures, which makes them difficult to classify.

One error is to presuppose the truth of an hypothesis, from which is made a prediction, and the outcome of the prediction is then used as support for the hypothesis. All too often, this support loses any provisos at first applied to it and comes to be presented as unqualified proof.

The word *hypothesis* is used loosely by medical writers to mean an idea, a guess, a theory, or a concept; whereas, as with all words, it has a precise meaning. An hypothesis must be consistent with what is known, and it must be testable (see p. 66). William Silverman[14] wrote of medical research, '"What is the question?" takes precedence over all other considerations. . . . A question should be considered genuine only if it refers to an hypothesis that can be overturned by defined events.' He went on: '. . . hypotheses to be tested must be formulated before examining the data that are to be used to test them.'

Unless medical researchers take care to think clearly and express themselves clearly, the formulation and use of hypotheses is an easy trap. The communicators of a study ought to know how the question was formulated; all readers can do is infer it from the report.

Another error of logic occurs when physiological studies are used to justify clinical practice, without measures of clinical outcome.[15] This error is often compounded by selectively ignoring factors not considered in the study.

These are not deliberate errors; the writers believe them, if only by repetition: 'What I tell you three times is true' (Lewis Carroll, *The Hunting of the Snark*). They are made more likely by the pressures to produce results and be relevant, and researchers may deliberately massage their data, but few of us have the ability to make deliberate errors of logic.

Senior doctors are not immune from errors of logic when they have preconceived ideas. An article and letter in the *British Medical Journal* signed by officials of British specialist societies expressed regret that because of changes in the career structure it would be more difficult in the future for junior doctors to do research. They assumed that a period in research is beneficial to all doctors as part of their training, and then supported their case by remarking on the large number of juniors wishing to take advantage of the opportunity. There was no mention that appointment committees demand, not knowledge of research method, but publications.

The desire to contribute to medical practice should not lead writers to draw unwarranted conclusions from what would stand alone as reasonable contributions to medical knowledge. Appointment committees and grant-giving bodies encourage these extrapolations when they ask, 'But what use is it?' The utility of the answer is something entirely different from the validity of the question.[14] The value of research to the novice researcher is learning the methods, which include clear thinking, clear language and clear exposition.

It is only an assumption that encouraging verbose, contorted language is more likely to cause logical errors, but surely this style does not enable clear, logical thought? 'Has the time not come to ask the writer(s) with ostensibly valid results simply to provide the busy working reader, the official beneficiary of this mammoth effort, with (a) the message and (b) the proof that the message is true, and do away with all the flannel?'[16]

Clear reasoning can be difficult in medicine, where dogma and entrenched attitudes are common, and where most clinical diagnoses are made by intuition. There is plenty of room for intuition in science and medicine, but not when drawing conclusions from clinical trials about treatments. The time for intuition is in the construction of the hypotheses, either as the primary questions asked in trials or as unanswered and further questions emerging from the results of trials.

Summary

If forced to list keywords to tag this discourse on the writing malaise we might choose:

- limitations
- imitations
- obfuscations
- specializations.

Limitations on the production of lucid writing are both real and perceived. The real include a lack of awareness, a failure of education and training, an absence of editorial guidance; these may be countered by practical solutions, such as we offer here. Perceived limitations are more difficult and more dangerous. They concern how writers interpret or decode the existing body of medicoscientific 'literature', and to what ends they use that personal interpretation.

Limitations of perception are inseparable from *imitations*, which themselves have simple and complex forms. Simple imitations provoke easy sympathy: 'I see and hear these [objectionable] forms of expression all day and everyday, and I cannot help but copy them.' But pushing the analysis soon reveals complexity: 'if my peers and superiors write in that way, then so should I [to gain respect, to succeed?]'. The matter of conformity is never far from the argument about 'good' and 'bad' writing, particularly when linked with the rhetorical 'objectivity' required of scientific expression (pp. 10 and 26).

Rhetorical analysis, we have said, is beyond our present scope, but linguistic analysis can be readily applied to medical writing. Consider those much-imitated 'hedging devices', which linguists have subjected to uncomfortable examination. A *Lancet* editorial,[17] aptly titled 'Trimming hedges', offers its first sentence for 'deconstruction':

> *It seems* [shield] that *most* [approximator] contributors to medical journals find it *extremely difficult* [emotionally charged intensifier] *to be certain which of their conclusions have been proven and which not* [passive voice], *or so one must assume* [(paradoxical) expression of author's personal doubt].

The article goes on to consider how far hedging is merely stylistic vagueness and how much 'a resource used to express scientific uncertainty'. We worry that such endemic *obfuscations* (*obfuscate* (*COD*): darken, obscure, confuse) are an intentional watering down of medical prose, almost as if there have been protective legal interventions. Some may consider this verging on the paranoid but, in a book review:[18]

> Another *disturbing* [our emphasis] problem . . . is the inability of some of its [the book] authors to resist making unreferenced statements that, however innocuous they may seem to anesthesiologists, may prove problematic when used against us by lawyers. . .

and in an 'Opinion' article in *Nature*:[19]

> . . .there are occasions when a scientific article may seem to readers to be damaging to established interests, perhaps those of medical practitioners or manufacturers.

Will there come a time when a medical piece goes to the 'legal department' before submission for publication? And might an apparently obfuscatory author have writs more in mind than writing (particularly when so much research is sponsored by commercial concerns)?

As to *specializations*, we are sure that the sort of objective lexical analysis described by Hayes[19] would confirm the anecdotal impression that the medical literature, because of the use of specialized language, is becoming increasingly obscure to all but 'initiates'. In commenting on 'the drift towards inaccessibility' in scientific writing, Hayes detects an obvious 'side-effect' of unrestrained language specialization:

> . . .that ideas flow less freely across and within the sciences, and the public's access to (and maybe trust in) science is diminished.

We have argued that public access is burgeoning via the Internet; it is the diminution of trust that remains an issue.

In a nutshell then, the darkest interpretation of the story so far is that medical writing in English is often bad to the point of dreadful. Its exponents, or certainly the younger ones, have passed through an increasingly restrictive and specialized system of education in which the placental nourishment of English literature is severed at a tender age. They then find themselves required, largely without formal guidance, to furnish evidence of their abilities – though one might ask, abilities of what? – by writing and having published academic papers. The models for these great works are their colleagues' academic papers, of variable quality, many of which have not been subjected to any significant editorial process whatsoever. In words that suit the topic: there exists the potentiality for an on-going vicious circle situation.

Of course, there are many doctors and medical scientists who write well.[2] We have tended to concentrate on poor writing because in medical science it is stereotyped and, therefore, easy to recognize, whereas good writing generally has the one quality: clarity. Compare two passages: the first from a specialist monograph published in America, the second from Sir George Pickering's classic textbook *High Blood Pressure.*[20]

> The broad indications for invasive measurements can properly be restated – that is; when the availability of hemodynamic descriptors complement the etiologic and functional diagnosis, define the likely temporal progression of the changing pathophysiology, and modify or may modify the therapeutic approach to management.

> As my scientific colleagues remark, the idea that a quantity, arterial pressure, has to be treated as a quantity and not arbitrarily divided into two ('normotension' and 'hypertension') is a glimpse into the obvious. Nevertheless, physicians of my generation, and even those of the rising generation, yearn for a definition of 'hypertension'; they clutch hopefully at every straw and even try to persuade themselves that the curve relating arterial pressure to mortality is composed of two linear relationships which cross at 140/90.

No doubt the writer of the first passage would agree with the one who wrote, 'A question is only interesting if there is a meaningful further discourse or procedure. Meaning is a property of statements that empathizes with the internal context of the understanding mind.'

Sir George Pickering, however, wrote further down the same page of his book that 'The function of language is to convey meaning', and we agree with him.

The ability to write clearly is a skill, not an art, and it is learned by practice. Most doctors will be active in research for only a few years of their careers. If they dismiss the writing up of their research as a necessary evil then they lose an excellent chance to improve their writing, and though they may never need to look at another experimental protocol, there will always be a need to write: to colleagues, to patients, to newspapers, to parish magazines.

The ability to write well is always useful.

PART II

Solution: symptomatic relief

3

Guidelines to clearer writing

Watson and Crick show how it's done

In 1953, Watson and Crick wrote a letter to *Nature* that must be one of the most important publications in the biological sciences.[21] It occupied just over one page of the journal, including the references and acknowledgements. It is a good example of clear scientific writing, and many of the principles of clear writing are well illustrated by their opening paragraph.

> We wish to suggest a structure for the salt of deoxyribose nucleic acid (DNA.). This structure has novel features which are of considerable biological interest.

Why is this a good example?

- It is direct. 'We wish to suggest. . .' not *In this communication is made a suggestion. . ..*
- It comes straight to the point. They could have started with a general statement about DNA: *Deoxyribose nucleic acid is a nucleotide that has been isolated from many species. We wish to suggest. . ..* To write this would have reduced the impact.
- They make two simple statements in two short sentences. They could have linked the sentences: *We wish to suggest a structure for the salt of DNA that has novel features that are of considerable biological interest.* This version is more clumsy and also ambiguous: it is not clear now whether it is the suggested structure, or the salt of DNA itself, that has the novel features.
- They are not afraid of using the same word, *structure*, twice. Many writers would have started the second sentence with a pronoun, such as *It. . .*, or used a synonym, such as *This configuration. . .;*

neither device would have been as effective as repeating *structure* (see THAT and WHICH, p. 132).

- Every word is necessary: 'We wish to suggest a structure for the salt. . .' not *We propose a possible structural hypothesis concerning the salt. . .*. They even avoid *molecular structure*, there being no other type of structure to which they could be referring. And, while most writers would probably write *We would like to. . .*, they use the elegant 'We wish to. . .'.
- Every word is the correct word, particularly *novel* (*COD*: of new kind or nature, strange, hitherto unknown). They write 'features which are of considerable biological interest' not *features associated with considerable biological interest.*

We appreciate that in offering this analysis of just two sentences we are making value judgements set against an 'internal standard' that is inherently subjective. Our concern is clarity of expression; others concerned with rhetorical studies and 'discourse analysis' have found the same sentences to be excellent examples of the proposal that 'scientific writing is a world of ironic understatement'.[4] This may be so, but we hope that medical writers will learn to handle simple language before they venture too far into irony. In the context of our discourse, even Watson and Crick's paragraph is not 'perfect'. *We suggest. . .*is shorter than 'We wish to suggest. . .', and *considerable* could be omitted. *Novel* was, at the time, a good word. Now, perhaps because of Watson and Crick, it is overused: almost 1% of all papers on Medline in 1992 had *novel* in the title, and this had reached 1.4% in 2004.

Whatever the rhetorical context, writers should communicate their ideas clearly without ambiguity or obfuscation (*obfuscate* (*COD*): darken, obscure, confuse). Readers should be able to understand a sentence on first reading, each idea following logically from the previous one. Words should be chosen carefully for their precise meanings, and readers should not be left to try to work out what writers are trying to say. Do not be forced to say to a critic, 'You know what I mean'; make it clear what you mean.

Every subject, be it computer science, geology or medicine, has its technical language. We write, for instance, of *cortical* and *medullary* bone. Except for technical terms, though, medical English is not a special kind of English. There is an example in Watson and Crick's letter.[21]

> We have made the usual chemical assumptions, namely, that each chain consists of phosphate diester groups joining beta-D-deoxyribofuranose residues with 3′,5′ linkages.

Or, from a medical textbook:

> The luminal surface of each cell has an apical protrusion covered with microvilli, and a single cilium emerging from its centre.

Both these sentences contain words that the layman would not understand, but in each the sense is obvious from the construction and needs only the definitions of the technical words.

This next example, by comparison, is a tortuous way of saying that, provided patients are continent, they have to empty their stoma pouches only once each night.

> It is common for the need to voluntarily evacuate the pouch to occur on one occasion nightly; more frequent defaecation interfering with the patient's sleep has not been encountered in our continent patients.

The writer of the next example is trying to say that medical teachers of undergraduates tend not to let students look after difficult patients.

> The study confirmed the hypothesis that clinical instructors of undergraduate medical students would choose instructional techniques limiting active student involvement in patient care activities when faced with problematical situations.

There is no need to write like this.

Planning

Writing starts with planning. If you are writing a standard paper for a medical journal, then the outline for your plan will be the usual Introduction, Methods, Results and Discussion. The Methods section is sometimes expanded to Patients and Methods, and Results may be Observations. Start by jotting down short answers to these questions:

1 What was I trying to do?
2 Why did I think it was worthwhile to do it?
3 How did I do it?
4 What did I show?
5 What do I need to stress?

6 What excuses do I need to make?

7 What is my message?

8 What would I like to do next?

Introductions usually start with the answer to 2: a *brief* review of important facts and references. Most introductions, when first submitted to journals, are too long; many of them stay that way. The last sentence or paragraph of the introduction should state the answer to 1.

'Methods' is the answer to 3. Make your notes in a logical order, describing things in sequence.

Your results or observations, question 4, must be stated as you measured or described them, not as you choose to interpret them. Use tables and figures if they will help readers; dense paragraphs of text interspersed with numbers make for difficult reading.

The discussion is the most interesting part to write, but knowledgeable readers – and referees – will take far more notice of your methods and results. By all means fly a kite or two in the discussion, but too much speculation will almost certainly antagonize referees. Be particularly wary of criticizing all previous work as inadequate while at the same time making what seem to you perfectly reasonable excuses for why your results were not quite what you wanted. Paradoxically, there is a dearth of robust and accurate criticism in many medical papers. One way that criticism is diluted or obscured by timid, over-diplomatic or inept writers is through the adoption of 'conventional' scientific style.

Keep in mind that 'What is the question?' (see p. 18 and Silverman[14]) is the single most important part of a clinical trial and, by extension, of any research. You should make sure that it remains uppermost in your readers' minds as they digest the fruits of your labours.

Getting started

The most difficult thing is getting started. You've done your research; you've bought this book; you've made some notes. Make sure you will be undisturbed – and get on with it! Your first effort will not be the final version, that is some way off yet; but the first effort is the most difficult.

Once your first draft is written, you can use this book to improve it, but it will help if you think about these four guidelines:

1 Prefer familiar words. Use the words you would use if you were discussing the work informally with a colleague. Unfamiliar words should become apparent if you put the first draft away in a drawer then re-read it a week or so later. It may help to speak the text into a tape recorder and listen to it later. This does not mean that that you should write exactly as you speak, but it may enable you to detect the more awkward sections of the text, particularly as speech is usually divided into smaller chunks than writing. If you obey guideline 1, then guideline 2 will follow.

2 Prefer short words in short sentences. Long sentences can confuse readers, who should be able to read through your article without constantly referring back. Longer sentences also make faulty constructions and incorrect grammar more likely. The corollary is to make every word count.

3 Get at least two people to read your article. If you really want help with the style and clarity, ask someone who is not a close colleague (perhaps someone with whom you do not always agree).

4 Read books about English. This book is a guide to the more common or important faults of medical writing. Our hope is that writers will be stimulated by it to take a real interest in the English language.

Some grammatical terms

This book is primarily about style, but poor style commonly contains incorrect grammar, so this book contains some discussion of grammar and grammatical terms. Grammar is divided into morphology, which is the structure of words, and syntax, which is the structure of sentences (i.e. the relations between words). The words *grammar* and *syntax* are often used interchangeably, and informally grammar is taken to mean sentence structure. We will use only the word *grammar*, although we are mostly concerned with style, which is a sort of subjective view of syntax: syntax with value judgement.

W. F. Whimster[22] wrote of grammar: 'I look at the grammar in a simple way – checking all verbs for their subjects; all pronouns for their nouns; all adjectives and adjectival clauses to see what noun they are telling me more about; all adverbs and adverbial clauses for the verbs they modify. . .'.

The simple definitions that follow, using the quotation from Watson and Crick on p. 25, should suffice. Other terms are explained in the text where appropriate.

A *noun* is a word that gives a name to something: 'We wish to suggest a *structure*. . .'. A noun can be represented by a *pronoun*: 'We [wish]. . .' represents the writers' names; '*which* are of. . .' represents features.

A *verb* is a word denoting action or being: 'We *wish* to suggest. . .'. Verbs can be *finite* – that is, have a subject, '*We* wish. . .' or '*which* are. . .' – or they can be *infinite* – that is, without a subject, 'We wish *to suggest*. . .'. In infinite form, verbs can act as the object of another verb – strictly the complement, 'We wish *to suggest*. . .' – or they can act as adjectives (the *suggested* structure) or as nouns (their *suggesting* of a structure). These last two forms of the verb are *participles* of the verb *to suggest*. Verbs have *tenses*, which indicate the time or completeness of the action.

An *adjective* describes a noun: '*novel* features. . .', '*biological* interest. . .'. An *adverb* describes a verb (for instance: this structure *certainly* has) or an adjective (for instance: *truly* novel features).

A *preposition* indicates the relation of a noun with another noun or noun equivalent (see below). Examples are *to, from, above* and *below*, but also 'features. . .*of*. . .interest'. The correct choice of preposition is one of the small things that have a large influence on style.

A *conjunction* links words or groups of words that have the same grammatical value. Some words, depending on the context, can be either prepositions or conjunctions. *As* and *since* can be prepositions, conjunctions or adverbs. Misuse of these small words is frequent in sloppy writing and is a common cause of ambiguity.

Phrases and clauses are groups of words. They can take the place of the various parts of speech, for example there are noun phrases and adjectival clauses.

A *phrase* is a group of words without a finite verb: '[We wish] *to suggest a structure for the salt of DNA*' is a noun phrase acting as the object, strictly the *complement*, of *wish*.

A *clause* is a group of words that includes a finite verb. A *main clause* makes sense by itself; a *subordinate clause* does not. 'This structure has novel features [main clause] which are of considerable biological interest [subordinate adjectival clause].'

Using a word processor

There are now few medical writers who do not use a personal computer and word processor, which makes altering draft typescripts much easier than it used to be. Once a terrible chore, making alterations is now almost too easy; writers – but particularly their supervisors – must be disciplined enough to prevent incremental improvements delaying the submission of a paper unreasonably.

All the more important to get it right first, or at any rate second or third, time – for which a word processor is of immense help.

Spelling checkers are useful provided they allow the addition of words not in their standard dictionaries, otherwise there will be an alert every time you type a drug name or unusual disease. Medical spelling checkers are now available commercially but are probably not worth buying by individuals. Spelling checkers are most useful for correction of typing errors such as *likley* for *likely*, or *hopsital* for *hospital*. Some programs, for example the almost ubiquitous Microsoft Word®, will correct these mistypings automatically. Annoyingly, this 'correct as you type' is usually the default setting, which is fine for correcting *likley*, but makes it difficult to type *likley* when you actually want to. It is sometimes better to work with automatic correction turned off, going through the document for spelling later, either accepting or rejecting the spelling checker's suggestions. Remember that *from* for *form* (or vice versa), and *fro* for *for* (*for* for *fro* is less likely in medical texts) will slip through, because they are all words. Spelling checkers, by their insistence on allowing only an initial capital, are also probably responsible for the loss of capitals in acronyms. AIDS is becoming Aids, which is fine half way through a sentence but a source of ambiguity when Aids is the initial word.

All word processors have a find command that allows the user to find a particular 'target' in the text. Most have a FIND AND REPLACE command that allows particular targets to be replaced. The exact instruction depends on the program but, if you want, for example, to change all spellings of *colour* to *color*, you can simply FIND [colour] REPLACE [color], which saves a lot of time.

We do not suggest leaving your word processor to undertake even apparently simple tasks unsupervised, unless you are an enthusiastic neologist. A colleague describes how the instruction just cited inadvertently created a new species, the 'Colourado' beetle. A labour-saving dodge for replacing '-ise' with '-ize' (these endings are not always interchangeable, see p. 69) produced, among other anomalies, 'milliseconds'. If replacing *colour* with *color* is part of revising a document to use American spellings, check whether there is an option to alter the preferred spelling between UK and US English (the default is almost certain to be US English).

Correcting style is largely a matter of pattern recognition: once you realize that *it has been noted as* is poor style, your eye will be caught by it as you read. If you know you have a tendency to use a particular marker of poor style – and it is easy to do so when hurriedly writing a first draft – then you can use FIND AND REPLACE to help you. FIND [with respect to] REPLACE [**with respect to**] will mark each occurrence of the phrase for your attention.

Many word processor programs also have grammar and style checkers, which 'must rank as the most ill-conceived products ever devised. It's not that all their advice is bad; it's simply that you can't pick out the occasional sensible comment from all the stupid ones unless you know your grammar. In which case, you don't need the grammar checker'.[23] They are getting better, but they are still infuriating, and infuriatingly slow. A sentence from above was run through a grammar checker.

> We do not suggest leaving your word processor to undertake even apparently simple tasks unsupervised, unless you are an enthusiastic neologist.

The program rightly picked up neologist, which is itself a neologism, and we invented it. Its grammar correction was to suggest that 'a missing *that* could cause confusion'. It could indeed: starting *We do not suggest that leaving your word processor. . .* is completely wrong. However, *that* might have been necessary if we had written *We do not suggest leaving your word processor to undertake even apparently simple tasks unsupervised is sensible, unless you are an enthusiastic neologist.*

The following convoluted passage scarcely worried the grammar and style checker at all.

> An analysis of practitioner cognitive activities in the context of a complex domain like anesthesiology, industrial process control or aviation is based on using knowledge about the cognitive demands of the task domain and data about practitioner activities to analyze practitioners'

information processing strategies and goals given the resources and constraints of the situation.

Only 'is based on' as a possible passive (see p. 139) was deemed worthy of comment.

This book will certainly help you to understand what grammar checkers are attempting to do. In the end, a knowledgeable human being is, with the recognition of good style that comes with practice, a far more efficient producer of good prose than a computer is.

Spelling

No one can pretend that English spelling is easy. French and Italian lose letters that are not pronounced but are otherwise phonetic. German and Welsh are phonetic. We marvel that those whose first language does not even use English characters ever learn to spell in English. There have been efforts over the years to simplify English spelling, but none has succeeded; nor will they – and nor should they, but this is not the place to present the arguments. English spelling of English may slowly lose out to American spelling, but that is a different matter. Bill Bryson writes of spelling reform (see the reading list, p. 242) that, 'It is hard to say which is the more remarkable, the number of influential people who became interested in spelling reform or the little effect they had on it.' According to George Bernard Shaw, the Irish playwright who on his death in 1950 left a bequest to help to reform English spelling, the letters *ghoti* spelled fish. The bequest had no effect whatsoever, and how ghoti spells fish is revealed at the end of this section.

Many spelling errors are typing errors that slip through despite the best efforts of writer, subeditor and computer spelling checker. The mistakes listed here are not uncommon. It can be a mark of illiteracy or carelessness (which we do not intend as judgemental terms) not to spell correctly; but we must acknowledge that many highly competent people cannot spell, perhaps because of dyslexia,[24] and their number may be increasing.

The following list of common problem spellings – indicated in the examples by [WRONG] – is not exhaustive.

-ABLE/-IBLE

There was no discernable [WRONG] difference between the groups.

Quite a few medical writers appear not to know which words end in *-able* and which in *-ible*. That incorrect versions sporadically get into print is the responsibility of (sub-) editors who, like writers, should be able to use spelling dictionaries. Of *-able* and *-ible*, the former is showing signs of neological dominance in submitted manuscripts. This may be because some writers also believe *-able* is capable of mating freely with any noun that has the temerity to lack this particular adjectival form. Inventions such as *pipettable* and *scanable* might just be acceptable as refreshing neologisms but the trouble is that these will inevitably reproduce themselves in more complex and ugly forms such as *scanability* (see also -WISE, p. 94).

ACCOMMODATION

Accomodation [WRONG] for the day surgery unit. . .

Accommodation: double 'c' and double 'm'.

ALRIGHT/all right

If nothing goes wrong – is everything alright? [WRONG]

Alright is not correct, but its use is increasing. *Alright* may eventually be accepted and distinguished from *all right* in the same way that *already* developed from *all ready*.

As in these examples, alright fits well in narrative.

> 'Every doctor except my GP said, "It's very serious," but they wouldn't say, "You're not going to die" or "It's an everyday operation." I kept being told, "You've got the best surgeon" but they couldn't tell me, "You'll be alright."'

> Subjective financial strain at T1 was assessed by asking: 'How well would you say you are managing financially these days?', responses to which were coded as: (a) living comfortably or doing alright; (b) just about getting by; or (c) finding it difficult or very difficult.

ANCILLARY, AUXILIARY, DOMICILIARY

Ancillary has only one 'i'. Auxiliary and domiciliary have the same ending.

BREACH/BREECH

> Yet this trial failed to adequately appreciate both the complex nature of vaginal breech delivery and the complex mix of operator variables necessary for its safe conduct. Widespread acceptance of this trial's results has breached the limits of evidence based medicine.

In consecutive sentences in the same paper, appear the correct spellings of *breech* (an archaic term for buttocks, as in riding breeches) and *breach* (meaning a gap). Doctors rarely used the word breach, except to misspell *breech delivery*, but it is currently one of the most feared medical words denoting, as it does, the failure to achieve government health targets.

> According to its own quarter end data, calculated in proportion to overall patient numbers, Newcastle had the sixth highest percentage of breaches in the country.

CAESAREAN/CAESARIAN

Choose one form and be consistent. Bryson and the *COD* go for Caesarean. Whether or not you use an upper or lower case 'c' in this instance, there is a preference not to capitalize modified or adjectival forms of eponymic medical terms: for example, Cushing's syndrome but cushingoid changes.

As Americans use the 'ce-' form (cesarian), there are eight ways of spelling the word.

COMPLEMENTary/COMPLIMENTary

> The Faxletter will be complimentary [WRONG] to our own Newsletter. . .

> Clinically relevant principles. . .are complimented [WRONG] by an outstanding art programme. . .

Complement to com*plete*. Both of these (the second from a publisher's advertisement) should be 'e' not 'i'.

> Professor Edward Ernst, chair of complimentary medicine at the University of Exeter, said he had heard anecdotal reports that the cyanide. . .

Whether or not there is a specialty of complimentary medicine, the chair is of complementary (non-allopathic) medicine.

CONSCIOUS

Has an 's' in the middle: it is not *concious*.

CONSENSUS

> Fortnightly Review: Concencus [WRONG] on diagnosis and management of primary antibody deficiencies.

This is a common error. Note that a consensus (one 'c' only) *is* a collective opinion (consensus has the same root as *consent* not as *census*): to follow consensus with *of opinion* is tautological (tautology: saying the same thing twice in different words). Similarly, *general* consensus is unnecessary.

> There was consensus between both groups that redundant publications occur because authors feel the pressure to publish.

There can be consensus within a group, but here *Both groups agreed. . .* will do.

> In contrast, formal methods of consensus development provide a means of managing group decision making so that all participants have the same influence on the outcome.

Consensus is correct, although it is a noun used as an adjective (see p. 162). At least the writer has not written the *group decision making process* (see p. 152) (in which *decision making* would also need to be hyphenated; see DEPENDENT below), but the sentiment expressed here is suspect: in what sort of group do *all* participants have the same influence?

COUNSEL/COUNCIL

To give psychological and social support is *to counsel*, by a *counsellor*.

DEPENDENT/DEPENDANT

> . . .transmittance waveform in the APTT coagulation assay is due to the formation of a calcium dependant [WRONG] complex of C-reactive

protein with very-low-density-lipoprotein and is a novel marker of impending disseminated intravascular coagulation. . .

Dependent is the adjectival form of the noun *dependence,* meaning reliance, the state of being dependent. A *dependant* (noun only) is one who depends on another. *Independent* has only the adjectival form, so does not behave in the same way.

Novel (see p. 77) is incorrect, and better simply omitted. An incidental feature of this quote is the confused use of hyphenation in 'stacked modifiers'. *Calcium dependent* as an adjectival complex is conventionally hyphenated *(calcium-dependent complex)* for clarity whereas *very-low-density-lipoprotein* contains a desperate excess of hyphens; *very low-density lipoprotein* is sufficient hyphenation for most tastes. Incidentally, adverbs ending in -ally do not need hyphenating to the following word: conventionally-hyphenated is wrong. Few writers would think a hyphen necessary in *completely emptied,* but it is a common error to write, for example, the grammatically equivalent *Formally-tested.*

DILATION/DILATATION

We agree with Bloom and co-authors,[25] who concluded a review of the etymology of these words by favouring the shorter *dilate* and *dilation.*

DISCREET/DISCRETE

Our team's programme doctor was as discreet as possible when contacting women about interviews. . ..

Discreet means prudent, unobtrusive; *discretion* is the noun. *Discrete* (the one more commonly used in medicine) means separate, individually distinct; *discreteness* is the noun. A way to remember the distinction is that the e's are separated in *discrete.*

It covers many aspects of arts interventions, including those where the boundaries become blurred, involving the usually discreet [WRONG] areas of architecture and interior design.

In this book review published in a medical journal, the point surely was that architecture and interior design are separate: discrete?

DOMICILIARY, see ANCILLARY

DRUG NAMES

The likelihood of misspelling drug names has increased with the European Commission directive on internationally approved non-proprietary names (INN). Eventually we will get used to them; many are no more than *ph* replaced by *f* (cefalosporins) or *th* by *t* (meticillin). Some are more radical (and controversial): *epinephrine* replacing *adrenaline,* for example.[26] Three drugs are worth mentioning because they are common drugs and commonly misspelt: *gentamicin* does not contain a 'y'; hydralazine has only one 'l'; and amitriptyline has only one 'y'. If you look on Medline, you can find versions of amitriptyline with just about any possible combination of 'i's', 'y's' and single or double consonants.

FOETUS/FETUS

The *COD* has *foetus* as the British and *fetus* as the American spelling. *Fetus* is becoming more common and some British journals prefer it for typographical reasons. Pick one and remain consistent: if the subeditors dislike your choice they will change it.

INOCULATION

> Unicef has also innoculated [WRONG] an estimated 25000 children against polio and measles in the camps. . .

Does not have a double 'n'. Unfortunately, innocuous does.

INTUSSUSCEPTION

We have to admit that this is a frightful word to spell (and it is not in my spelling checker's standard dictionary). It seems more logical that it should begin *inter-*, but it doesn't; then there is the double 's' and remembering where the 'c' goes.

IT'S/ITS

> The EMO system: it's [WRONG] origins and development
>
> . . .a capnometer with it's [WRONG] breath-through cell. . .

It's is the shortened form of *it is* and nothing else, despite popular pressure to the contrary. Unlike nouns in possessive constructions (the surgeon's knife; the patients' prescriptions) the possessive *its* (belonging to the family *his, your, their*) does not have an apostrophe. Nor does *hers*, and although neither of us has seen *her's* in a medical text the error did appear on the medical page of the *Independent* newspaper of 27 March 1990:

> The treatment is expensive (her's [WRONG] cost £3000) and is still being evaluated.

A further comment about the possessive apostrophe is more appropriate here than in the section on punctuation: what to do about names that end in s. Is it Jones' or Jones's findings? The best advice is to go with the pronunciation: so Jones's findings, St James's Hospital, but Gowers' *Complete Plain Words*.

Despite the number of hospitals in which notices read *Childrens Ward* and *Womens Health*, these need apostrophes, which, because the nouns are already plural, are placed before the 's': *Children's Ward, Women's Health*. If the noun has been made a plural by the addition of the 's', the apostrophe is placed after it: *Technician's Room* for one technician; *Technicians' Room* for more than one.

Apostrophes sometimes intrude into plurals (the famed greengrocer's apostrophe, *apple's and pear's*, and locally to one of us, *fish n'chip's*). Letters about apostrophes appear sporadically in the correspondence columns of daily newspapers. A wonderful example was a letter about a baker selling 'gateaux's'. Taken from the same language, a roadside sign for an inn declared 'A'la carte menu'.

An apostrophe is not needed when referring to years, as in: *The work was done in the 1970s. . .*, but this is a point of style about which a minority of publishers disagree.

LEAD/LED

The past participle of the verb *to lead* is *led*: a mistake that can slip past even the sharpest of eyes.

LITIGIOUS

This is a word that we may, unfortunately, (see p. 21), come to see more often in medical texts. There is no 'n'.

> . . . obstetric patients are potentially more litiginous [WRONG] possibly because they [have a] high expectation of a satisfactory outcome

MIOSIS/MEIOSIS

Miosis is constriction of the pupil; meiosis is a type of cell division.

MUCOUS/MUCUS

Mucus is the noun, *mucous* the adjective: the membrane is a *mucous membrane*. On the internet search engine Google Scholar, *mucous membrane* won 17 600 to 566 over *mucus membrane* (a ratio of 31 to 1), so this is a common misspelling even among those who should know. On plain Google, the ratio of correct to incorrect was halved (313 000 to 19 300: 16 to 1).

Mucosa is (*COD*) a mucous membrane, whose plural is mucosae.

NAUSEOUS/NAUSEATED

Bryson counsels that *feeling nauseous* is wrong because nauseous means *causing nausea*. He prefers *feeling nauseated*. However, according to the *COD*, *nauseous* means either *affected with nausea* or *causing nausea*. The dictionary *Merriam-Webster OnLine* says that those who insist that nauseous cannot mean affected with nausea are wrong, because it is the most common use of nauseous. To us, *nauseating* seems a more natural adjective for something that causes nausea, but the divergence is probably one between American and UK usage.

Both dictionaries list *nauseousness*, an entirely unnecessary alternative to nausea.

OCCURRED

> If this effect occured [WRONG] in cancer surgery. . .

> This occured [WRONG] in spite of. . .

There are rules governing what happens when endings such as *-ed* and *-ing* are added to words. The general rule is that the consonant doubles if the preceding vowel is written with a single letter *and* that vowel is stressed.

Thus *occur* becomes *occurred* (and *prefer* becomes *preferred*) and *benefit* becomes *benefited* (and *vomit* becomes *vomited* – and *vomiting*, not *vomitting* or even *vommitting*, which are common spelling mistakes in clinical notes).

> At the end of last month, the union ballotted [WRONG] its members
> on strike action. . .

Ballot (as in voting) becomes *balloting* (with the emphasis on the first syllable in both words). *Ballott* (as in palpating kidneys) becomes *ballotting*, with the emphasis on the second syllable.

The letter 'l' is doubled after a single vowel in UK English even if the vowel is unstressed, thus *travel* and *travelled* (but unusually *parallel* becomes *paralleled*). The 'l' ending does not double in American English: thus *beveled*, *labeled*, *traveled* are correct in the USA. In Canada, 'the more "up-market" the readership, the more British the spelling; the more popular the readership, the more American the spelling' (*Reader's Digest Guide*: currently out of print). We leave writers intending their words of wisdom for the Canadian journals to decide for themselves on the height of their market.

Focus can become either *focused* or *focussed* (*OED*) but there is a general preference for the former. But see FOCUS.

As there are exceptions to these rules, and American spelling is different in other ways as well, writers should use a good dictionary (such as the *Oxford Writers' Dictionary*) to check what happens with a particular word. There is a section in Fowler's: *doubling of consonants with suffixes*.

American usage affects meaning as well. When Britons and Americans use completely different words for the same item, such as when referring to water taps or to faucets, this may puzzle but generally does not confuse. It is when the same word has subtle but important differences that problems may arise. The *pavement* in Britain is where you walk; in the USA it is the surface on which you drive. The urgent advice 'Get onto the pavement!' could have disastrous consequences. In both countries, *momentary* means *lasting for a moment*; but whereas *momentarily* means *for a* moment in UK English it means *at any* moment in American English. British doctors off to conferences in America need not worry when American pilots announce that the aeroplane will be taking off momentarily. Confusions of meaning are not usually a problem for medical

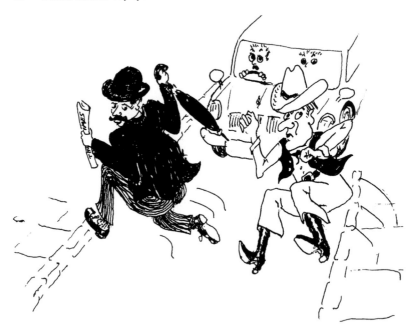

Get onto the pavement!

writers, but remember that *presently* means *in a short while* in UK English but *at the current time* in American English.

OPHTHALMIC

Ophthalmic has two 'h's. It is often spelt wrongly as opthalmic. Perhaps there is confusion with *optic.*

PRACTICE/PRACTISE

. . .too far divorced from their parent discipline to practice [WRONG] it. . .

The noun is *practice;* the verb is *practise.* Think of *advice* and *advise.* This is so for *licence* and *license* also: *his licence licenses him to do animal work. . ..*

This is not so in North America, where *practice* and *license* are the correct forms for both noun and verb, but our examples are not from American writing.

. . . a urologist practiced [WRONG] in the art of endoscopy.

Urologists need to *practise*, but probably consider endoscopy a skill rather than an art.

PRINCIPAL/PRINCIPLE

> . . .beef products are . . . the principle [WRONG] remaining candidates as a source of human infection. . .

These two have different meanings; they are not interchangeable. The main thing is the principal thing; main and principal both contain an 'a'. A principle is a rule; rule and principle both contain an 'e'. These statements don't make much sense, but may make it easier to remember which is which. The usual mistake is the one in the example; principal for rule is less common.

PROSCRIBE/PRESCRIBE

To proscribe is to prohibit or denounce. There is nothing wrong with the word, but a typographical error can easily change it to prescribe, readily overlooked during proof-reading.

RESUSCITATION

Try remembering this as pronounced 'resus*k*itation'.

USING CAPITALS

Doctors often use unneeded initial capitals: Urology, Intensive Care Unit, Orthopaedic Surgeon. Interestingly, patients and nurses are less likely to have capitals than Consultants and even Specialist Registrars. In German, all nouns have capitals; in English, only proper nouns do so. The increasing use of acronyms (see abbreviations, p. 188) in everyday language (UNESCO, NATO) is probably partly to blame for the increase in initial capitals, but current editorial policy in many English newspapers and magazines has greatly diminished initial capitals as a mark of (over-) formality, which is to be welcomed. Specific institutions wear capitals better than the generic terms: so *the Smith Orthopaedic Hospital did 426 hip replacements last year,* but *hip replacements are better done in specialized orthopaedic hospitals.*

> [This is] a time when the issue of inequalities in health is being sidelined. For conservative social commentators such sidelining is a component of general propagandising against equitable redistribution of income. . .

Someone who is conservative is not necessarily Conservative; and these social commentators were Conservative but definitely not conservative.

A particular bacterium, such as *Staphylococcus aureus*, has a capital 'S' (even if shortened to *Staph.* or *S.*) and the genus/species binomial is usually printed in italics, but the general terms staphylococcus and staphylococcal have the lower case and are not italicized (see also CAESAREAN).

A PUZZLE

Ghoti spells fish because gh is pronounced as in tough, o as in women, and ti as in nation.

4
Is there a better word?

A medical writer, when asked why he had used the words 'were haemorrhaged' instead of 'were bled', replied that he thought *haemorrhaged* was more scientific. Sometimes we do need to use a term more precise than the one in common usage, but *bled* is a perfectly good word, and *haemorrhaged* tells us no more about the process. (*Haemorrhaged* is also incorrect grammatically. *To bleed* (*COD*) can be transitive or intransitive, in other words may or may not have an object: you can bleed someone to death, or you can yourself bleed to death. *To haemorrhage* is intransitive and so cannot have an object: you can only bleed to death yourself; you can't haemorrhage someone else to death.)

During *Alice's Adventures Through the Looking Glass*, the birds held a meeting.

> 'In that case,' said the Dodo solemnly, rising to its feet, 'I move that the meeting adjourn, for the immediate adoption of more energetic remedies –'
>
> 'Speak English!' said the Eaglet. 'I don't know the meaning of half those long words, and what's more, I don't believe you do either!' And the Eaglet bent down its head to hide a smile: some of the other birds tittered audibly.

Resist the urge to use words that are less familiar. There is danger that the unfamiliar will contribute to confusion; or to put it another way, inflated language often sets out to confuse. Most of the words in the lists that follow can be replaced by words that are more common.

English is a rich language that has many roots, which makes it particularly rich in synonyms. Synonyms rarely have precisely the same meaning; by using the less familiar word, you may give your writing an unwanted shade of meaning, or sometimes the chosen word is wrong (see Hayakawa and Ehrlich, Reference books, p. 240). Francis Crick[27] wrote of the danger of choosing a word for what you think it means, when he chose *dogma* to describe a proposed mechanism in genetic theory: 'As it turned out, the use of the word dogma caused almost more trouble than it was worth. Many years later Jacques Monod pointed out to me that I did not appear to understand the correct use of the word dogma, which is a belief *that cannot be doubted* [Crick's italics.].' Jacques Monod was French.

Do not use a word because you think it 'sounds good' – unless you know what it means – or you will appear not scientific but foolish, as in these two examples.

> Ideally the wound suture method should augment the short stay surgery.

Augment (*COD*): to make or become greater.

> There were no differences in the anthropomorphic data. . .

The writer was comparing the ages, weights and sex ratio of the control and test groups of patients. *Anthropometric* (*anthropometry* (*COD*): measurement of the human body) is probably the intended word. *Anthropomorphism* (*COD*) is the attribution of human form or personality to a god, animal or object (see DEMOGRAPHIC).

Or you may appear pompous, as in this example:

> High frequency venturi jet ventilation is a recently perceived and appreciated form of mechanical ventilation.

Michael O'Donnell (see Reference books, p. 240) invented the term Decorated Municipal Gothic to describe this style of writing.

Alternative words

In the following, **against a word indicates a common fault. The most frequently abused and most easily replaced words are: *administer* for *give*, *demonstrate* for *show*, *employ* or *utilize* for *use*, *encountered* for *found*, *following* for *after*, *notes* for *noticed*, and *regime* for *regimen* or *scheme*.

**ADMINISTER*/give

This is one of the most common of the substitutions of long words for short. *Administer* is better used for its primary meaning of *the managing of affairs.* Use *give* unless either there is something very complex about the way a drug is given or the discussion includes the way that the drug is prescribed, prepared and given to the patient.

> Fentanyl was administered intravenously. . .

> Midazolam. . .was diluted. . .and administered through a centrally placed venous catheter.

> These [heparin, washed red cells and platelets] were administered because of recurrent severe anaemia. . .

Given is better in all three examples, although in the first *injected* could be used. *Injected* is certainly preferable for substances 'administered' under skin or into buttocks.

> . . .an infusion of dextrose saline was administered overnight. . .

> . . .a non-irritant drug that can be administered into peripheral veins. . .

Given is also better here, but even better is a more precise word: . . .*dextrose saline was infused*. . ., *a drug that can be injected*. . . .

> Sites of administration often implicated in extravasation injury include. . .

This was from an article about the complications of intravenous infusions. There are three points of style: *administration, implicated,* and *extravasation injury.* As the topic of the article was self-evident, *sites of administration* can be shortened to *sites. To implicate* is (*COD*) to lead to as a consequence or an inference; to show (a person) to be concerned in a charge or a crime. This is not the sense intended by the writer of this article. If you place a cannula too near a joint, then extravasation is more likely, but *implication* has connotations of intent or of a degree of complexity.

In the phrase *extravasation injury,* the noun *extravasation* is used as an adjective (see NOUNS AS ADJECTIVES, p. 162).

Try: *Extravasation causing injury often occurs if a cannula is sited near*. . . but we suspect the writer simply meant *Harmful extravasation often occurs after cannulation close to.* . . .

A D O P T/use

> Some radiologists will not adopt the small bowel enema because. . .

Use is almost always good enough although the sense here could be that some radiologists *do not like* using a small bowel enema. *Adopt* has the sense of *choose* or *take over*, which might have been meant here. If so, it could be the technique rather than the enema itself at issue and more not fewer words would have been needed.

ADVOCATE/suggest

Advocate (*COD*): plead for, defend; recommend, support (policy etc.). Do not use *advocate*, which implies a certain strength of feeling, if you mean merely *suggest*:

> Recently…angioplasty has been advocated as the treatment of choice for renal artery stenosis (Smith *et al.*).

The sentence reads more easily if one avoids the passive construction *has been advocated* in favour of the active *Smith et al. suggested angioplasty as the best treatment. . ..*

ADUMBRATE/outline

Adumbrate (*COD*): represent in outline; faintly indicate. Prefer *outline*. (See OBTUND)

AETIOLOGY/cause

Aetiology is (*COD*) the 'science of the causes of disease', not the cause itself (see METHODOLOGY, PATHOLOGY, TECHNOLOGY). It does not get used much for its strict meaning ('When is the next aetiology class? Is the teacher a trained aetiologist?') so perhaps it is not surprising that we say *The aetiology was unknown* when we should say and usually mean *The cause was unknown*. When overused, *aetiology* is a flagship of medical pomposity; using it does not get round ascribing causation (see Variations of BECAUSE, p. 128). In the right place, *aetiological* is perfectly acceptable because it has the meaning (*COD*): 'assigning a cause or reason'. The American spelling is *etiology*.

> The aetiology of delusion of pregnancy is likely to be heterogeneous.

Sometimes cause is unknown; sometimes there are too many possible causes. *Heterogeneous* (composed of parts of different kinds, and well applied to a group of patients some healthy and some suffering one of a number of different diseases) is not a synonym of *multifactorial,* which is meant here. Note that the ending of heterogeneous is *-eneous,* not *-enous.* (*Heterogenous* syn. heterogenic is a different word with specific meanings in biology and genetics. Similarly, *homogeneous* (the opposite of heterogeneous) and *homogenous,* a word meaning genetic homology.)

AFFORD/give

Local injections often afford complete but temporary relief. . .

Give, or *provide,* is better.

ALLUDE/refer, mention

The misuse of *allude* for *refer* is not so common in written medical English but is ubiquitous in meetings and spoken presentations. An *allusion* is an indirect reference. When a speaker has described treating urinary tract infections with amoxicillin, it is incorrect then to say, 'When you alluded to amoxicillin. . .'; the speaker *referred to,* or even simply *mentioned.*

> Each poster bears a sentence in fine print pointing out a disease whose elucidation or treatment has materially benefited from animal research, and whose features are alluded to by a pun in the main slogan.

Allude is correct: the pun is an indirect reference.

> At this point I mentioned Macmillan nurses and I quickly saw the patient's wife become uneasy. . . while he had not seemed to bat an eyelid when I alluded to Macmillan nurses, his wife was upset. . .

Allude is incorrect. *Mentioned* is probably best (but to save repetition in this sentence one could use 'spoke of').

ALIQUOT/SAMPLE

. . .investigated by analysing sequential 2 ml aliquots of 10 ml samples.

Aliquots of 1 ml arterial blood were drawn 5 times. . .

An *aliquot* (*COD*) is a part contained by the whole an integral number of times; a *sample* (*COD*) is a small, separated part. The first example illustrates the correct usage; the second example is incorrect.

Aliquot is anyway an overworked word and some journals debar it, even when used correctly (which it rarely is). If *sample* has already been used to describe the major part (as in the first example), *portions* or even *sub* (-) *samples* will do for the further divisions.

AMELIORATE

. . .it often takes longer for the hypertension to be ameliorated. . .

Some longer words are just plain clumsy. *Ameliorate* means (*COD*) to (cause to) become better; Gowers prefers *improve*, but that is not correct here. Nor is *alleviate* (to make less burdensome or less severe), another word often better replaced. When hypertension is treated, the blood pressure decreases, and *lessen*, *settle*, or *resolve* is suitable, depending on the sense and if you are inhibited in using the efficient but colloquial *get better*.

Worsen is often better than *aggravate* or *exacerbate*.

AMOUNT/NUMBER

The amount of people predicted by the year 2000. . .

Amount refers to mass; when referring to people use *number*. Amount is to LESS as number is to FEWER (see p. 70): so balding people have a smaller amount of hair, which consists of a smaller number of hairs.

APPROXIMATELY/about, almost, nearly

Pancreatic cancer affects approximately 6000 people in the United Kingdom every year

Average reported daily intake of heroin was approximately 0.75 g

Approximately four weeks later, as the effusion had not resolved, the joint was explored

This deterioration occurs because *P falciparum* undergoes repeated cycles of maturation approximately every 48 hours

If it is more or less that number, which is so for all these examples, *about* is better. The *Penguin Guide to Synonyms* (Hayakawa and Ehrlich, Reference books, p. 240) is strict about *approximately*, which 'implies an accuracy so near to a standard that the difference is virtually negligible'. We prefer *almost* negligible to *virtually* negligible, and we like the distinction from the less precise *about* but fear that approximately, being satisfyingly polysyllabic, is now a true synonym of about.

If the sense is a number not quite achieved, then the words *almost* and *nearly* are better than *approximately*.

ARMAMENTARIUM/drugs, treatments

(*COD*) The medicines, equipment and techniques available to a medical practitioner. Doctors love this word! Especially in lectures: how it rolls off the tongue. Mostly it is either a tautology or wrong. Most commonly it is a pompous replacement for 'drugs'.

> . . .From antibiotics to tube feeding, the professionals have an armamentarium of treatments to keep the very old and infirm alive a few days longer. . .

The armamentarium *is* the range of treatments. If armamentarium is the wanted word *of treatments* should be omitted. Otherwise, *range* or *wide range* is better; simply *many* is enough.

> . . .Our therapeutic armamentarium is limited to the more tried and tested generic drugs of proven efficacy. . ..

If armamentarium means all available treatments, then we suppose that *therapeutic armamentarium* is a valid description of all available drugs. But *We are limited to. . .* is neater and means the same.

> . . .conventional magnetic resonance imaging is only the first of an array of methods that will eventually comprise the NMR diagnostic armamentarium.

This example is not helped by the misuse of *comprise* for *make up* (see p. 54). *Armamentarium* and *comprise* can both be bypassed by *that will eventually use NMR in diagnosis*.

> As none of the older neuroleptics are as effective or free from unwanted effects as we would like, risperidone is a welcome addition to the pharmacological armamentarium.

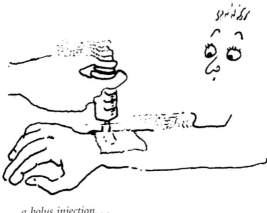

. . . a bolus injection. . .

Coming towards the end of an editorial, this sentence loses nothing by losing its last four words. Remember *none* takes the singular (see p. 146).

AUTHOR/worker, investigator

These authors proposed that. . .

The proposition was made consequent on a scientific study to which the writing was incidental (what are we saying!). *Workers* or *investigators* are better words. Don't forget there can be easy ways of dropping these descriptors altogether. The example is from a sentence that followed one in which 'These authors' were named in a reference. Thus *They proposed that. . .* would be understood.

BOLUS/injection

The strict definition of a *bolus* (*COD*) is a large pill or food at the moment of swallowing. This definition does not cover the injection of a drug. However, this is a useful new meaning of the word if used to describe rapid intravenous injection. It is particularly useful when injections are being given at the same time as an infusion of the same drug. There is a tendency to overuse *bolus* as an adjective (*bolus injections*), and often it is better replaced by *rapid*, or left out.

BULK/most

What is not clear is how the bulk of the care can be shared most satisfactorily and effectively between the general practitioner and the community midwife.

The bulk of should be applied only to mass or volume not to number: *the bulk of the care* is correct (care having abstract volume); *the bulk of the patients* would not be (see MAJORITY).

Although *the bulk of the care* is syntactically correct, the whole sentence is turgid and it is not clear why *the bulk of the care* is referred to specifically. Try *It is not certain how best to share the care between the general practitioner and the community midwife*, or a little more colloquially *How best is care to be shared. . .?* Medical style is often refreshed by posing questions more straightforwardly as questions, however rhetorical. The late J. R. A. Mitchell chose a question as a title to an excellent, and well written, review[28] of the treatment of heart attacks: 'Back to the future: so what *will* fibrinolytic therapy offer your patients with myocardial infarction?' The title was designed to attract more readers than the dull alternative *A historical perspective of the treatment of myocardial infarction.*

CAPABILITY, CAPACITY/can

Writing that X has the *capacity* or *capability* to affect Y is an inflation; *can* is what is meant. In speech, *capability, capacity* and *can* may be stressed to hint that the quality in question, though existent, is not always operative. In writing, this nuance is not possible without explicitness or (in fiction) the skilful elaboration of context. In scientific writing, *can* without further qualification best means 'can and does'. If the intended meaning is 'can but doesn't always' or 'can but only if. . .' this should be stated.

***COMMENCE, INITIATE/BEGIN, START*

Begin, start, commence, initiate? In general, use the word that you would use in everyday speech; this makes *start* and *begin* preferable to *commence* and *initiate. Initiate*, with its overtones of religious rites, is a poor choice. The overuse of *initiate* has attracted the same overuse for *initial*, now commonly used adjectivally as a turgid way of saying *first*.

COMPARABLE/SIMILAR

The groups were broadly comparable with respect to age and weight.

In a clinical trial, the only difference between the control group and test group should be the treatment under study. For this, the groups must be *comparable* (capable of being compared), so features of the groups other than the difference in treatment should ideally be identical. This is impossible, but they must be *similar* (resembling but not the same).

In other words, this example means that *the groups were comparable because their ages and weights were similar*. It is better expressed as *The groups had similar ages and weights* (see WITH RESPECT TO).

Strictly, any one thing is comparable with any other, however bizarre or odious the outcome. *Comparable* is widely abused as a way of side-stepping *similar*. This may be because the items under comparison were not quite as alike as was hoped for. And using *similar* correctly provokes the sometimes uncomfortable question, 'How similar?' whereas *comparable* has a looser, less provocative feel to it.

COMPRISE/are, make up

There are few published data to show that specialist centres do any better at treating the common adult cancers of breast, bowel, and bladder that comprise the routine workload of peripheral hospitals.

The cancers *are* the routine workload.

One could equally ask: who comprises the Resuscitation Council?

Comprise is incorrect (see below), and *makes up* may be correct, but it depends on the sense: *are* is correct if the question is *Which organisations are responsible?*; *is on* is correct if the question is *Who are the individuals?*

**COMPRISE/CONSIST, include

Comprise means *consist of*, so *Treatment comprised bisoprolol, captopril and a diuretic* and *Treatment consisted of bisoprolol, captopril and a diuretic* are both correct. Our preference is *consist of*.

Do not use *comprise* if there is only one item: *The anticonvulsant comprised diazepam; was* will do.

> . . .complications comprising of hallucinations and involuntary movements. . .

Comprise means consist *of,* so *comprise of* is incorrect. Perhaps some writers are thinking of *composed of.* Using *comprise* or *consist* implies a whole that is made up of a number of parts. Complications are not a whole; new ones may be described subsequently: *complications including. . .* is better.

> This was a consecutive series comprising all patients presenting between. . .

Here *comprising* can be omitted: *This was a consecutive series of all patients. . ..*

> In 1977 accidents with baby walkers comprised 13.5% of accidents that involved. . . transport devices.

Comprise is incorrect. *Of accidents involving* (or better, *with*) *transport devices, 13.5% were with baby walkers, x% another device and y% another device.* One of the types of accident (those with baby walkers) cannot comprise or consist of part of the whole (accidents with transport devices). A comprises B, C and D; B, C and D are each a part of – but cannot comprise – A. Replacing *comprised* by *made up* or *accounted for* is correct.

CONCEPT/IDEA

Concept is a word beloved of advertisers ('A new concept in designer kitchens') and best avoided in serious writing. Bryson wrote, 'If all you mean is "idea", use "idea".'

> Quality of life is a difficult concept to define.

Idea is better, but neither word is necessary; it is quality of life, not the idea of quality of life, that is difficult to define.

CONSTITUTES/is

> The examination of urine specimens constitutes a major portion of the work of a clinical microbiology laboratory.

This sentence contains three ill-chosen words. *Constitutes* (*COD*: make up, be the components of) is better replaced by *is*. *Portion* is a word better applied to food; *part* is just right here. MAJOR (see p. 113) should be replaced by a more precise word: do the writers mean it is an important part of the work or a time-consuming part?

CONSTRUCTED/made, designed

The model was constructed using the principle described by earlier workers. . .

Constructed is usually better replaced by *made*, though in the example, about a theoretical molecular model, *designed* is better. Use *constructed* if nuts and bolts, or plastic and glue, were used to put the thing together, otherwise *made* is simpler and less pretentious (see also USING).

CONSULTED/asked

Consulted implies advice has been asked of an expert. *Consultant* and *consultation* obviously have particular meanings in medicine.

DATA/information, RESULTS

Data are the observations or measurements made in the course of a study. It is a word best applied to numbers and, particularly in descriptive work, *information* or *results* may be better. However, *results* as in *Our results show. . .* should not be allowed to displace the richer *Our findings are. . ..* Results come directly from actions taken (tests made, experiments conducted) whereas findings are part of a broader scientific process of observation and reflection. *Outcome* is a useful substitute for *result(s)* in some contexts.

Data is a plural noun (but see p. 148); for a unit of data, *datum* (the singular) can be used, especially for computed quantities. The commonly seen *data point* is both incorrect (it should be *datum point*) and, more important, tautologous.

Another common phrase is *raw data*, used to mean the experimental measurements before any transformation or analysis. If they are the measurements, then refer to them as measurements.

**DEMOGRAPHIC

The demographic data, ages, weights and gender, are shown in Table 4.1.

Demography is (*COD*) the study of statistics of births, deaths or disease as illustrating the conditions of life in communities. The ages and weights of small groups of patients admitted to clinical trials are not demographic data. There is no simple single word to use instead but that is no reason to use a word that has a clear and entirely different meaning. If all that are included are the ages, weights and sex of the patients, refer to them as such. In the appropriate contexts *baseline characteristics*, *physical characteristics*, or *anthropometric data* may be correct. The phrase *patient data* is common. It is ugly (see Nouns as adjectives, p. 162) but better than using *demographic* inappropriately. (See also GENDER.)

**DEMONSTRATE, EXHIBIT/SHOW

The results. . .demonstrate that the. . .ventilator has been modified. . .

Intravenous urography demonstrated that the tumours were all large. . .

Reserve *demonstrate* for an active illustration (a working model, an experiment in front of an audience, a computer simulation); otherwise use *show*. *Exhibited* is another pompous substitute but endemic in clinical medicine, where patients endlessly exhibit their diseases (but attract no buyers). *Exhibit* has the same unnecessary theatricality as *display*, as does *present with*. The use of *When a patient presents with*. . . to mean *When a patient is first seen and has*. . . is of some merit (and we certainly don't expect it to disappear) but the effective word *presentation* in obstetrics is probably where this usage should have come to rest.

DISINTERESTED/UNINTERESTED

The specialist journals are filled with papers written out of necessity and read with disinterest.

The first and proper meaning of *disinterested* is 'impartial', distinctly different from 'uninterested' (lacking an interest in), but the two are now used almost interchangeably. From our example, it might be said that it is the *referees* of scientific papers who *should* be disinterested; readers may well be uninterested in 'papers written out of necessity'. Here, *without interest* is better.

Disinterest is probably a word to avoid: few people now know that disinterested can mean impartial. You are likely to be misunderstood if you claim that to be disinterested is a virtue. Write impartial, unbiased or neutral.

> Hardly any serious, financially disinterested commentator would now argue that we should move to a system based on the American. . .

Impartial is better.

> The 1990 contract forced disinterested general practitioners to collect meaningless data and to hold health promotion clinics. . .

The general practitioners were uninterested.

> Simple semantics may help quell patients' fears that they will be seen by a scruffy, disinterested youth who may well later report their intimacies in the bar. . .

Again, the feared youth is uninterested, although reassurance will probably help more than semantics. In formal writing, *help* should be followed by *to*: thus *Semantics may help to quell . . .*

EFFECT/AFFECT

I effected the treatment means *I carried out the treatment*. *I affected the treatment* means *I had an influence on the treatment*. Writers sometimes confuse the words:

> Does the position of the probe effect [WRONG] the results. . .

Alex Paton[29] wrote 'these words are commonly used, and misuse may seriously affect (alter) meaning' and gave an example:

> Consequent development of the act is *effected* [his italics] by the requirement of central government to produce five yearly plans for primary health care services.

Paton commented, 'Do they really mean that or has someone got a letter wrong?' Single letters can be important (see PRESCRIBE).

EFFICACIOUS/effective

Efficacy has a precise meaning in pharmacology relating to the maximal effect of a drug at a receptor. If writing simply of treatment of diseases *effective* is better.

> . . .ritanserin was efficacious for a period of six weeks.

A *period of six weeks* is six weeks (see p. 155).

ELEVATED/ENHANCED, *increased*

> . . .and enyzme levels gradually became elevated. . .

To *elevate* is to bring to a higher position, literally (*an elevated section of railway line*) or metaphorically (*elevated from bishop to archbishop*). *Raised* may be a better and simpler word for the literal meaning and is used in medicine (*a raised, erythematous rash*). The step from specialist registrar to consultant is merely promotion, not elevation. In the example, *gradually increased* is better (see LEVEL). Beware also of *remained elevated*; remained raised is better.

Enhance has the sense of intensifying. Unless this is the sense you want, increase is better.

These words often form expanded verbs: *the drug caused an increase* or *the drug resulted in an elevation* instead of the simpler *the drug increased. . .* (see p. 154).

EMPIRICAL

Empirical has two meanings (*COD*): based on experiment, not theory; and deriving knowledge from experience alone. Taking the first of these meanings, *We must collect empirical evidence* means that we have an important scientific experiment to do. Taking the second, *They have only empirical evidence* is a criticism that anecdote is not enough for scientific proof. As its meaning depends entirely on context and point of view, empirical is best avoided altogether (see Brewin[30]).

> Empirical self-treatment of travellers' diarrhoea was pioneered in the early 1980s.

This meant treatment without evidence of the identity of the infecting organism. It could just as easily have meant the opposite. *Self-treatment before definitive diagnosis of travellers' diarrhoea was pioneered...* is longer, but is not ambiguous.

A *British Medical Journal* editorialist wrote that 'The recommendation... is not based on any evidence but is purely empirical'. An editorialist in the journal's family member, the *Journal of Medical Ethics*, was at the same time announcing the launch of 'Empirical medical ethics'. Unlike the usual brand of ethics based on theoretical discussion, this was actually a series of observational medical ethics. Ethicists really should be more careful with words; even for their observations, words are all they really have.

**EMPLOY/use*

Gowers writes of *employ*: 'Prefer use if that is what you mean.' *Employ* has connotations of payment and it is rather silly to think of employing a gastroscope or a gas flow.

> ...the range of fresh gas flow which is normally employed in clinical anaesthesia...

This means *the usual range of fresh gas flow*.

> ...when very small volumes are employed...

This can be rewritten *when small volumes are used* but better still is *when the volume is small.* (See VERY.)

**ENCOUNTERED/seen, found, OCCURRED*

> Resistance encountered during the insertion of the tube should alert the user...

To encounter means *to come across*, as in one's travels. In that sense, the example shows correct usage because one does 'come across' resistance when inserting tubes or cannulae. The sense is unaltered if encountered is deleted – unless one wants to stress that the problem is with the tube rather than with the person inserting the tube.

> Leakage of saline from the device as encountered in *x* cases...

As encountered in can be replaced by *occurred in*, but we suggest this less confidently than in the first edition of this book. 'Occur' and 'occurrence' have risen in the scale of overused words in medical writing. They are frequently superfluous and can be replaced by more direct statements. It seems to us that the notion of an 'occurrence' has become invested with almost mystical 'objectivity'. We have seen the awful phrase 'occurrences of recurrences in relation to metastasis'.

> . . .the aetiology most likely to be encountered is that of trauma. . .

To be encountered is superfluous; so is *that of: the most likely aetiology is trauma. . .* (but see AETIOLOGY).

EPOCH/PERIOD

> Measurements were made over epochs of five breaths. . .

An *epoch* is the beginning of an era in history, or a period in history or life marked by special events. It is also a specific geological term of time. As five breaths are unlikely to take more than 20 seconds, *epoch* is not the best choice of word here. There may be need for a word other than *period* if there is risk of confusion with period's mathematical meaning of *wavelength measured in units of time* (and beware the unnecessary use of *period*, see p. 155). *Segment, section* or sometimes *episode* can be useful to apply to experimental records. *Windows*, used metaphorically, is possibly an apt description of consecutive or even overlapping segments of experimental record.

EXIST(S)/are (is)

> . . .there exists a direct casual relationship between tumour recurrence and transfusion.

Exists is a pretentious substitute for *is*. If we give the writers the benefit of the doubt, *casual* may have been a typing or transcription error for *causal*: a direct casual relationship is a contradiction in terms (see RELATION).

Why not write . . .*transfusion makes* [or *may make* if you are not certain] *recurrence more likely?*

> . . .would allow a fresh gas 'buffer' to exist in the expiratory tubing. . .

Omit *to exist:* . . .*would leave a fresh gas 'buffer' in the expiratory tubing.* . . is then better.

> The solutions fill a hiatus that exists between crystalloids and blood products.

The word *hiatus* is no better than *gap*. But where is this gap? On the shelves in the casualty department? 'Sloppy language', Michael O'Donnell wrote, 'is a form of sloppy thought'.[10] Doctors write of existing hiatuses 'thinking they are adding dignity to their prose'. When what you want to say is *the solutions have properties between those of crystalloids and blood products*, then hiatus is not adding dignity, though it may provoke ridicule.

The pretension of *exists* appeals not just to medical writers. A hotel, being upgraded for the modern age, had this notice on display:

> The management is presently considering the existence of the snooker table.

EXPLORE/study, investigate

> Another aspect of crevicular fluid biochemistry explored in this study was the relationship of IgG, IgM and alpha-2-macroglobulin to that of prostaglandin.

Explorers explore; medical scientists study or investigate. *Biochemistry* is obvious and therefore superfluous, which does away with the awkward adjectival use of *crevicular fluid* (see Nouns as adjectives, p. 162). *Relationship* is imprecise; if we assume the quality of relationship is the amounts of the substances then try: *We also studied how the concentrations of IgG, IgM and alpha-2-macroglobulin in crevicular fluid correlated with prostaglandin.*

EXPECTORATE/SPIT

He expectorated into a handkerchief is not a polite way of saying that he spat: *to expectorate* means to eject secretions from the lungs or throat; *to spit* means to eject material, for instance saliva, food or blood, from the mouth.

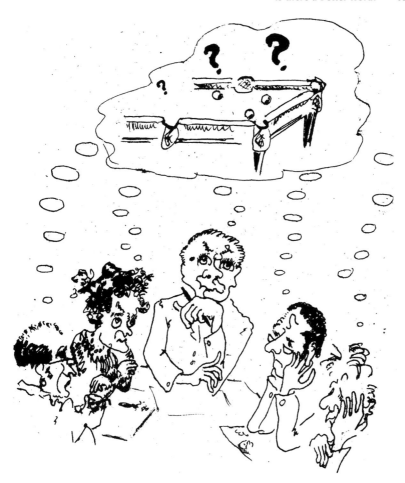

The management is presently considering the existence of the snooker table.

FATALITY, MORTALITY/DEATH

Fatality and *mortality* are sometimes the appropriate words, but more often they can be replaced by *death*.

. . .failure may lead to fatality.

Better as . . .*failure may cause death.*

For example, a fatality occurred when the flow of a pump was increased. . .

A patient died is better (unless it was the operator of the pump who died)

> . . .fire victim mortality.

Better as . . .*death caused by fire* (see Nouns as adjectives, p. 162). The dismal duo *morbidity and mortality* are tolerable as a label for statistical data but try substituting *illness and death* in ordinary writing. This sort of change simplifies and enlivens most texts. It would also bring some immediacy to clinical case conferences to describe them as *illness and death* meetings. This appeared in a case report in the *British Medical Journal*: 'She did not undergo treatment because of her age and multiple medical comorbidities.' It means no more than *we did not treat her because she was old and very ill* but, if you want to be more descriptive, *her many other diseases* is better.

FEASIBLE/PROBABLE/POSSIBLE

These words are similar but distinct. Something is *probable* if it is likely. Something that is *possible* is something that may happen, or that could happen if the circumstances were right.

Feasible, like *possible*, is more tentative than *probable* but has connotations of practicality: *the operation is feasible* (it is technically possible); *his idea is feasible* (it fits with what we know).

FOCUS/concentrates

Light is focused to a point and eyes focus on an object but investigators and their studies concentrate on the topic of study. The shorter word is not always best: the expression *to pay particular attention to* can be useful here (see TARGET).

> Within the medical and midwifery professions concern has been focused on. . .

There is no need to write of focusing concern. *Within the medical profession* means *doctors* (see Chapter 11 Circumlocution). Try *Doctors and midwives are concerned that. . . .*

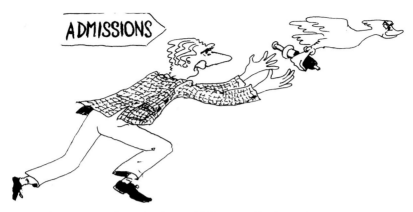

The man was admitted to hospital following a blood sample.

**FOLLOWING/after, because of

A blood sample was taken following application of a tourniquet to the upper arm.

Gowers describes *following* as a pretentious substitute for *after* and all the books listed in the bibliography condemn it (see also PRIOR TO). The example should read *A blood sample was taken after application. . ..* This misuse of *following* can cause ludicrous ambiguity: *The man was admitted to hospital following a blood sample.* This nonsense illustrates what *following* is: an active process.

If *following* replaces *because of* it can cause the same ambiguities as the use of SINCE.

GENDER/SEX

Bryson writes, '*Gender,* originally strictly a grammatical term, became in the nineteenth century a euphemism for the convenience of those who found "sex" too disturbing a word to utter.' Do not use gender when you mean sex: six men and three women is a *sex* ratio of 2:1. Gender often applies to chosen sexual expression: a male-to-female transsexual is of male sex but of female gender.

**HE/SHE/THEY

There were 15 men and 19 women included in the study. . . . . .he was asked to fill in a questionnaire about the preoperative visit.

The nurse had no difficulty operating the equipment, and he/she could give advice to the patient.

The policy of the *British Medical Journal* is 'to neutralise sex biased language. . .but we hope that authors will now start to do this for themselves'.[31] Writing *he/she*, though awkward, is better than referring to 19 women – a majority in the study – as *he*. (S)he is used by some. The best solution is to use the plural if possible: *Nurses had no difficulty. . .and they could give advice. . ..* *He/she* is a common use of the lazy slash (see p. 178). Our publishers advise, 'use him/her' or 'them' rather than 'him' (but we prefer that you rewrite to avoid excessive use of him/her).

A number of simple texts and papers have been prepared on this subject and it is essential that the author preparing his first manuscript should avail himself of these.

This advice, perhaps written with tongue in cheek, came from a medical journal's *Guide to Contributors*! *Authors preparing their first manuscripts* is an improvement but the advice becomes more direct and less stilted if rephrased: *There are a number of simple texts and papers on this subject, and authors preparing their first manuscripts should consult them.*

HYPOTHESIS/*guess*

An *hypothesis* is consistent with what is known and is testable; it is not a synonym for an *idea* or *notion*, which are more general terms. *Guess, speculation* and *suggestion* are all less formal and less rigorous terms than *hypothesis*. It is not uncommon to read in the Discussion sections of papers *We hypothesize that our results differ from those of Smith because. . .*; *suggest* or *think* is better. (See also CONCEPT.)

ILLUSIVE/ELUSIVE

. . .there are several articles that relate to the illusive problem of developing selectively toxic therapies. . .

An *illusion* (and hence illusive) is something that is not really there, for example a mirage. Something that is difficult to find is *elusive*, the word required here.

INCIDENCE/PREVALENCE

Incidence and prevalence have specific meanings in epidemiology and we urge that these be adhered to in usage that is even remotely epidemiological.

> There is discussion about the increased risk of dementia in elderly depressed patients. . .. The number of cases here is too small to [compare] with the expected population incidence, or with the incidence reported in previous studies.

The number of patients who have a disease or, as here, having one disease also have a second disease is the *prevalence*; the *incidence* is the number of new diagnoses of a disease per time. Prevalence *is* a rate; it must be quoted per number in the population:

> The validity of comparison between prevalence rates quoted in other studies is often difficult. . .

It is the comparison, not the validity, that is difficult; the difficult comparison affects the validity: *It may not be valid to compare prevalence between studies*, or *It is difficult to compare prevalences. . .*

INFER/IMPLY

Writers imply or suggest; readers infer or deduce. Implication, suggestion, inference and deduction can be done only by humans. Writing *These results suggest that. . .*, although very common, is technically incorrect, but likely to survive.

> Indeed, what is thought to be the original medical use of the word in the phrase 'the stroke of God's hand' inferred that this affliction was beyond earthly comprehension.

The medical use of the word *implied* that strokes could not be understood.

IMPACT/EFFECT

> This cutting back of resources is bound to have an impact on services.

> The impact of screening on the natural history of the disease is uncertain.

Impact implies physical contact, usually by heavy objects with one another or the ground. In both examples *effect* is better; in the second, *influence* is the best word. *Impact* is often used to emphasize that the effect is substantial (see p. 00), but in these examples, explicit description is more effective.

> *If we are not given the resources, then we cannot supply the service.*

> *We do not know whether screening will allow earlier diagnosis or alter prognosis.*

The verb *to impact* means to press or fix firmly in or into. The past participle is used in *an impacted wisdom tooth* or *there is a piece of meat impacted in the oesophagus*. Do not use *to impact* when you mean *to affect*; managers are often guilty of this misusage. Americans tend to use *impact on* to mean *have an effect on*.

> **This clearly has a negative impact on quality of life.**

A sentence which, when read, certainly makes life less worth living – and illustrates how difficult it is to describe the direction when *effect* or *impact* are used in this way. Returning to the first example, we infer that cutting back resources will make services worse, but we can express this explicitly only by writing of *a negative impact*. Sometimes, whether the effect is good or bad is not obvious:

> **These findings will have an effect on the service.**

Much better to say what is expected: the findings will improve, or worsen, or slow down or encumber. If the effect is unknown, then say so: *an unknown effect on the service*.

INFORMED/based

> **. . . comments informed by prejudice rather than reality.**

The phrase *informed by* is common, especially when referring to evidence gathered for an official report. It says no more than *based on*. The usage has led to *inform* as a transitive verb, the evidence *informing* the report. This is confusing and ambiguous because we generally regard the object of inform as *the person informed*: *he informed me of the evidence*.

**INITIATE, see COMMENCE

-ISATION/-IZATION, -ISE/-IZE

Phythian (*A Concise Dictionary of Medical English*: currently out of print) wrote that 'hospitalisation means no more than sending to hospital, and is uglier.' This is true, although the ugly one is in the *COD* and the *OED* comments 'Freq. commented on as an unhappy formation'. Certainly you should avoid inventing words by adding endings (see -ABLE/IBLE and -WISE), unless you are so confident of their value that you hope to find fame as their originator.

> We therefore performed a retrospective study of all patients entering our dialysis programme over a 4 year period, and studied survival and need for hospitalisation in relation to a number of factors.

We think hospital admission, despite the use of hospital as an adjective (see p. 162), is better, but hospitalization is here a marker of poor writing. Try: *We surveyed all patients who had entered our dialysis programme during the four years, relating survival and need for hospital treatment to a number of factors.*

> . . .she agreed to be admitted for lateralisation [of a tumour]. . .

Better as *to identify which side the tumour was on.* . . or *to localise the tumour.* . . – which must include determining the side. But:

> When the diagnosis is established, localisation of the tumour is essential prior to surgery.

This is ambiguous. Does the sentence mean that the surgeon has to know where the tumour is? Or does it mean that there must be treatment to reduce the extent of the tumour before surgery?

Whether a word ends in *-ise* or *-ize* is sometimes a source of confusion. In UK English, the two endings have come to be more or less equally chosen alternatives in common usage, except where *-ise* is invariable as in *advertise, excise, exercise* and words ending in *-vise* (such as *revise, supervise*). Many publishers favour *-ize*, where there is a choice, possibly because some dictionaries, including the Oxford, do so too. The *Oxford Writers' Dictionary*, an authoritative work, is comprehensive in choosing *-ize*. You should follow your publisher's, or journal's, preference if one is stated and attempt to standardize your piece to one or other form. Remember that words ending in *-(l)ysis* (such as *analysis, haemolysis*) become *(l)yse* (*analyse, haemolyse*) in UK English; *analyze* is correct North American usage.

In writing this book, we have reproduced in our quotations the endings chosen by their originators because quoters are obliged to reproduce the original precisely as it first appeared. In reforming a quotation, we have stayed with the originator's chosen ending but in our own text we have opted for *-ize* where there is a choice. The book therefore appears not to be 'standardized' but inadvertently illustrates a difficulty arising from a rich etymological heritage.

**LESS/FEWER*

Less surgical and more medical infections.

This was the headline of an editorial in the *British Medical Journal*. It should have read *Fewer surgical and more medical infections*.

Less and *fewer* are not interchangeable. *Less* is applied to mass; *fewer* is applied to number. A guide to using the correct word is to remember that *less* is derived from *little*, and *lesser* is the equivalent of *smaller*. Do not use *fewer* unless the item is notionally divisible into smaller units: balding men have *less* hair but *fewer* hairs; eat *less* sugar by having *fewer* spoonfuls in your tea. One can speak of *less surgical infection* [singular], but it must be *fewer surgical infections* [plural] – the sense intended in the example.

The drug causes less serious symptoms. . .

Grammatically, *less* can be an adjective or an adverb, *fewer* is an adjective. Thus *less serious symptoms* are symptoms that are less serious; *less* is an adverb qualifying the adjective *serious*. The writer meant that the drug caused fewer symptoms that were serious, and should have used *fewer*. This is an example of a small error having potentially serious consequences.

Sometimes, as in the next example, the potential ambiguity of *less* cannot be resolved without changing the word order.

We prefer to use less invasive monitoring

Does this mean *we prefer monitoring that is less invasive* or *we prefer less of the invasive monitoring*? This ambiguity would not occur in speech, when the meaning would be given by the stress.

The least rises occurred following mastectomy. . .

If rises *occurred less often* after mastectomy then *fewest* is needed. *Least* would be correct if the rises that followed mastectomy were *the smallest rises* – but may be misinterpreted (incorrectly) to mean fewest. *Smallest* is unambiguous and the better choice.

Less than half the sessions fall into the category. . .

The writer has taken *half* as singular. Here, though, the sense is of *a number of sessions*, and *fewer* is correct.

Defining and categorizing, putting things into groups and under headings, is fundamental to all research. Once the categories have been defined, it is better to write *Less than half the sessions are in the category. . .* than to use *fall* metaphorically, or you risk the guffaws that greeted the unfortunate registrar who announced at a research seminar, 'Grossly obese patients often fall into this group.' (See Metaphor, p. 156).

More risks the same confusion as *less*. *The drug causes more serious symptoms* should, according to sense, be written *The drug causes symptoms that are more serious* or *The drug causes additional serious symptoms*.

**LEVEL/concentration

The rate at which the plasma potassium level is rising is more important than the absolute value.

Levels of liquid rise and fall but the correct word here is *concentration* and concentrations of ions increase and decrease (see p. 154).

The *concentration of potassium in the plasma* is more elegant than the *plasma potassium concentration* (see Nouns as adjectives, p. 162). It is accepted usage to leave *concentration* understood; most journals will accept *The rate of increase in the plasma potassium. . ..*

LITERATURE/published work

In a survey of the literature from 1970 to 1987. . .

What niggles about this common usage is a nuance with at least two parts. First, medical writing is not really literature, one of whose meanings in the *COD* is writings whose value lies in beauty of form or emotional effect. It

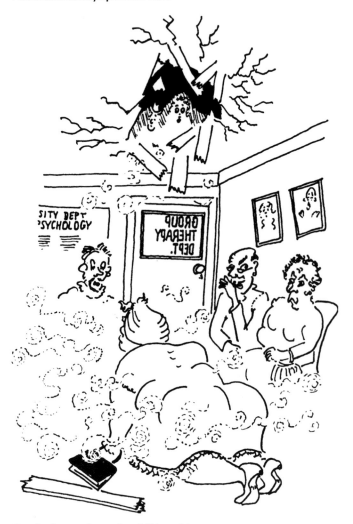

Grossly obese patients often fall into this group.

is a bit of a travesty to refer to reports of clinical trials and the works of Milton with the same word. *Published work* or *account* or *record* need have no connotations of beauty.

Secondly, the meaning of literature is generally more abstract than actual. Saying, 'Have you collected the literature on your planned holiday?' is a colloquialism where literature is reduced to meaning a pack of brochures. A *literature survey* is usually a schematic, itemized search of papers and books, not a philosophical overview of the subject (though the need to formulate the overview may be the reason for the search). In this sense 'the literature' is equivalent to holiday brochures and ought not to be referred to in more inflated terms.

> The previous literature in this area has focused on Crohn's disease presenting with anorexia nervosa.

The investigators, not the literature, do the focusing (see FOCUS). *Topic* or *subject* or *disease* is a more precise word than *area*; if a less precise word is wanted, *field* is better than area. *Previous workers in this field have focused on. . .* Note, though, that *previous* is unnecessary in either version because literature must already be in print, and the past tense (*workers. . . have*) has the same implication (see p. 150).

LOCATION/place, site

> . . .the optimum location for an intravenous infusion. . .

Optimal is better than OPTIMUM. *The best site* is neater; site is a shorter word.

**MAJORITY/most

> The vast majority of the responses were assessed by. . .

Most or *almost all* will do; *the vast majority* is unnecessary. Another example, 'The vast majority of obese patients. . .', conjures up a strange mental image (see BULK).

MALODOROUS/smelly

> Initial distress is compounded by that associated with a fungating and malodorous tumour mass.

Using *malodorous* as a polite euphemism for *smelly* distances readers from the patient's distress. *Initial distress is worsened by a fungating, smelly tumour* is direct and involves readers in the patient's predicament. *Tumour mass* means no more than *tumour*.

MANDATORY/ESSENTIAL

A fast-running intravenous infusion is mandatory.

Mandatory (required by law) should be replaced by *essential* (exceedingly important). The more direct *There must be a fast-running intravenous infusion* is even better.

More studies from different groups are mandatory to confirm [these] findings.

The studies are not required by law; are they even *essential*? It is more likely that they are merely needed: *Confirmatory studies are needed.*

Authors seem to think that *mandatory,* like PARAMOUNT, invests their writing with authority.

MAY/MIGHT

When used in the future sense, there is no difference between *may* and *might*: *There may be a pandemic of influenza* and *There might be a pandemic of influenza* mean the same. The subtleties of difference come when used for describing past events, when *might* has more of a sense of finality than *may.*

The dishonesty of the butcher at the centre of the outbreak of *E. coli* food poisoning may have contributed directly to the deaths of 6 of the 21 victims.

This is correct: it is still possible that the butcher was responsible, but we do not know.

If the outlets had been identified and the information acted on, the deaths may have been prevented.

This is incorrect: it should be *might* because the action can no longer be taken.

MAXIMIZE, MINIMIZE

Do not use these to mean merely *increase* and *decrease. Increase to a maximum* often means no more than *increase.*

MEANINGFUL

Meaningful can be replaced by *useful*, or omitted.

> The number of cases here is too small to make a meaningful comparison with. . .previous studies.

The opposite of meaningful is meaningless. If a comparison is meaningless, it is not a comparison: *The number of cases is too small to allow comparison. . ..*

> A more meaningful question is whether these disorders can coexist.

A better question is. . ..

METHODOLOGY/method

Medical workers have more than a passing interest in *methodology* (the science of experimental method) and its study would constitute a more feasible discipline than AETIOLOGY. But when they write they 'have adopted a new methodology' they mean they *have used a new method* and nothing more.

> Nevertheless, there are several general problems in assessing the trial evidence from guidelines. . . the methodological quality may not be discussed: although there are limitations of scoring systems, most back pain trials have low scores for their methodology.

Methodological is correct: the writers' interest is the study of method. But each trial does not have a methodology, and *methodology* at the end of the example is better as *for the quality of their methods* (which is reasonably contracted to *method quality*).

> Their findings, that up to 80% of acute hospital interventions had a scientific rationale, produced much comment and a challenge from the authors to repeat the study in other clinical settings. By applying the same methodology we investigated the degree to which general practice is evidence based.

> These methodologies have included repeated measurements of blood pressure using the traditional technique, self measurement of blood pressure in the home or workplace, and ambulatory blood pressure measurement using automated devices.

Methods is better for the first example, and *techniques* for the second.

MODALITY/method

Other treatment modalities had been exhausted.

Other *methods of treatment* is better, although the single word *treatments* is probably enough. People and supplies become exhausted, but treatments only fail; try *Other treatments had been unsuccessful.*

Proprioception and fine touch are examples of *sensory modalities*, a correct medical usage.

MODIFY/change

. . .the ventilator has been modified into a pressure generator.

To modify is *to alter slightly*; what is needed here is the more radical *change* (*the caterpillar changed into a moth*). Things *are modified*, they cannot *be modified into* other things: *. . .the ventilator has been modified* [implying a small physical alteration to the ventilator] *to make it a pressure generator.*

MONITOR/measure

From its meaning of a device (*COD*) for checking or warning about a situation, a monitor is (*COD*) any tropical lizard of the genus *Varanus*, supposed to give warning of the approach of crocodiles. Do not use *monitor* if crocodiles are unlikely and you simply mean *measure*. To monitor implies an action will be taken if a measurement is outside some range of normal: blood pressure is monitored in the intensive care unit but merely measured on a patient's routine admission to hospital.

MORPHOLOGY/SHAPE

The morphology of the electrocardiogram was unchanged means that the shape was unchanged. Morphology (like AETIOLOGY, METHODOLOGY, TECHNOLOGY and, to some extent, PATHOLOGY) is one of those words where the science or study of something has become confused with the thing itself.

**NOTED*/noticed*

Writing in the passive voice (see p. 139) often forces writers to use *noted*. *Noted*, meaning *written down*, is also used instead of *noticed*, meaning *brought to attention*.

> During the first 23 months it was noted that stomach cancer was very rarely associated with liver metastases. . .

Substituting *noticed* for *noted* gives the correct use, but this is still poor English – see ASSOCIATED WITH, VERY.

NOVEL/new

Novel means more than *new*: it means something of a new form or nature; something previously unknown. Watson and Crick[21] rightly applied it to the double helix, but these days it is used indiscriminately for things that sometimes are not even new (see p. 26).

OBTRUSIVE/obvious

> Other less obtrusive sources. . .

Obtrusive (*COD*): unduly noticeable. *Obvious* (*COD*): open to eye or mind, clearly perceptible.

ON-GOING/continuing

> This is an on-going investigation.

Why not *The investigation continues*, or *The investigation is not finished*? Perhaps this is another symptom of the contraction of language that eschews small words and active verbs in favour of strings of qualifiers (See Nouns as adjectives, p. 162): 'a small word and active verb eschewment language contraction symptom', perhaps.

OPTIMUM/best

OPTIMIZE/improve

Optimum is a noun as well as an adjective, so it is better replaced by *optimal* when used as an adjective. However, *best* is simpler. The verb *optimize* is often an incorrect substitute for *improve*: optimize means (*COD*) make the best or most effective use of.

OBTUND/suppress

OBVIATE/prevent

Obtund and *obviate* are better replaced by the simpler *suppress* and *prevent*. What is the attraction of these words – another is ADUMBRATE for *outline* – over the simpler alternatives? They may be impressive to some English readers, but to foreign readers they are likely to be confusing. There are entries for *obviate* in Cassell's French and German Concise dictionaries, but not for *obtund*. *Adumbrate* appears in the French, but not the German.

PARADIGM/example, pattern

> Periodically it is necessary to reformulate scientific explanations in the paradigms of the time.

Paradigm is a grammatical term, overused as a synonym for example or pattern. If you wish to put forward new ideas in scientific understanding, writing of *reformulating in paradigms* is not only incorrect but is more likely to confuse than to clarify.

Thomas Kuhn[32] used *paradigm* as a 'term that relates closely to "normal science"'. By this definition, scientific explanations *are* the paradigms of the time.

> Conference. The challenge of breast cancer: Treatment: How far has the contemporary paradigm taken us?

Paradigm is meaningless. We do not even know what it refers to: is the paradigm our current treatment, or our current understanding of the disease? An example of how clear thinking, which is needed for better understanding of disease, is hindered by language.

> The paradigm of medical decision-making has been shifting in recent decades, from physician dominance to patient participation.

The paradigm of can be omitted, but even then the sentence is a poor way of writing *Patients now have more control than formerly over their medical treatment.*

PARAMETER/VARIABLE

Parameter has a precise mathematical meaning; it is not a synonym for *variable* or *measurement*. Nor is *parameter* synonymous with *limit, boundary* or *condition*, though that does not stop politicians using *parameter* for all of these. *We have to look carefully at the parameters of health care* is completely without meaning. *Paradigm* and *parameter* share the characteristic of 'impressive overuse'.[33]

If you measure the heights of each in a group of patients, height is the variable, not the parameter, being measured. If the distribution of the variable is normal, i.e. Gaussian, the mean and standard deviation are the *statistics* that describe the sample. They can then be compared with the *parameters* of the distribution, which are the mean and standard deviation of the population from which that sample is drawn (see p. 194).

Incidentally, *statistics* as a branch of mathematics, or as a word, takes the singular (*statistics is not an easy subject for many doctors; statistics has three syllables*); the statistics of a particular study takes the plural (*the statistics are complicated*).

> We noted the following parameters: time of closure of colostomy, presence of radiological leak, histological differentiation. . .

Should be *variables*, though *the following parameters* can simply be omitted.

The distinction between parameter and variable is less clear when deriving more complex values than simply the means and indices of variability of the measured variables – for instance, measuring the changing plasma concentration of a drug with time in order to define the pharmacokinetics of the drug: volume of distribution, elimination half-life, clearance, and so on. These are pharmacokinetic *parameters*: the parameters that determine the concentration of drug in the compartments of the body.

In the equation of a straight line $y = mx + c$, x and y are variables, m and c are parameters, and thus the following is correct:

> For the population biologist, behavioural alterations count if the parameters of the equation vary.

> . . . it is important that the patient be given the truth about the parameters of treatment available . . .

We applaud the correct use of the subjunctive – that the patient *be* given the truth – (see p. 96), but what does *parameters* mean? We cannot know without the context. Types is the most probable meaning, but costs, consequences and side-effects are just some of the possibilities.

> For every increase of 20 mmHg above normal the pH falls by 0.1; for every decrease of 10 mmHg below normal the pH rises by 0.1. Any change in pH outside these parameters is therefore metabolic in origin.

The word needed here is limits – which is the commonest general meaning of the word.

> . . .you must receive the treatment within the parameters of the clinical trial in question.

According to or *defined by* is probably best.

> If consent has been obtained, this tissue should normally be used in preference to tissue for which the parameters of consent are inadequately recorded.

The ethical issues of consent are tricky, which makes the words used by those discussing them even more important than usual. Not only is it unclear what the parameters of consent are in this sentence, it was equally unclear in the article from which the sentence was taken.

In computing, a parameter is a variable that is passed to a subroutine.

PATHOLOGY/disease

Pathology does not mean *disease* and should not be used as a synonym (see SPECTRUM). However, *pathology* has become accepted as *symptoms of a disease* (OED) or *the sum of morbid processes . . . in a specific disease* (Butterworth's *Medical Dictionary*), which makes the distinction between *disease* and *pathology* less clear.

PARAMOUNT/foremost

This vogue word emerged at the time of the Falklands conflict in 1982, when the Prime Minister Margaret Thatcher talked of the wishes of the Falkland islanders. Mostly, it is a pretentious way of saying *foremost*, and sometimes what is described as paramount is no more than important. As the word tends to be used by those with a vested interest, it is best avoided (see also MANDATORY).

**PERFORM*/carry out, FUNCTION*

'If you mean no more than *do*, then that is a less misleading word to use.' (Gowers) *To carry out* is a better verb to apply to ordinary actions than *to perform*, as in this example from an editorial:

> Every day endotracheal intubation is carried out many thousands of times in anaesthetic rooms throughout the country. . .

Function is a better word than *perform* to apply to the working of an organ of the body. This example is stilted:

> . . .to know how the kidney will perform. . .

Replacing *perform* with *function* improves the style; better still is *to know the renal function*. (But see FUNCTION, p. 98.) *Perform* is commonly superfluous – a consequence of constructions that use the passive voice (see p. 139).

PERSONNEL/staff

The simple word *staff* has been usurped by the longer, and we think more impersonal, word *personnel*. The impersonality of *personnel* is a resonance from the proper distinction of meaning between it and *staff*. *Personnel* (*COD*: a body of persons employed in public undertaking, armed forces, etc.) is the original opposite of *matériel* (*COD*: available means, esp. materials and equipment in warfare). *Staff* is (*COD*) 'a group of persons carrying on work under manager etc.'. Both personnel and staff are collective nouns taking a singular verb (see p. 147).

But even personnel is better than its later replacement *human resources*, which prompted a columnist[34] to write that it is 'an expression that

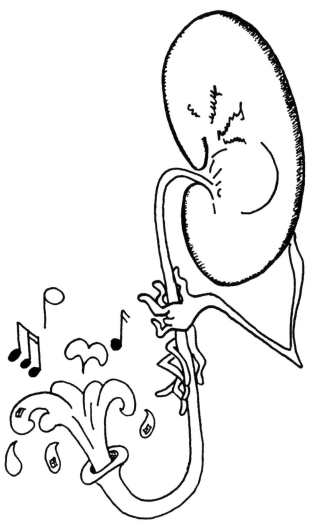

. . .to know how the kidney will perform . . .

inspires in me nothing but gloom. It speaks of a management world view in which employees are on a par with electricity.'

POPULATION/SAMPLE, *group*

The treatment was effective in this elderly patient population.

We recommend precautions are taken for this hypertensive population.

Population has probably gained a hold in this context by attraction – from its use as a statistical descriptor. The population is all those people living in a village, town or country. To write of an elderly population or a hypertensive population implies that the people in the village, town or country tend to be elderly or hypertensive. Unless that is what you mean, sample or group is probably the correct word: *The treatment was effective in this group of elderly patients.* For the second example, *population* is best replaced by *patients*: *We recommend precautions are taken for these hypertensive patients.*

> Despite the small population sample. . .

Despite the small sample. . .

> The study population consisted of female patients . . . admitted consecutively to the acute wards. . .

Again the correct word is sample, but better is simply *We studied all the women admitted to the acute wards. . ..*

Note that only things that are whole (like a fruit cake) can be divided. Populations are whole and can be divided into groups; groups are whole and can be divided further. If a population or group has been divided into categories then *sub(-)set* is an alternative word. Patients are not whole and it is better to write of patients being *allocated* to groups.

POSSESS/have

> The third generation cephalosporins possess a number of desirable properties compared with the earlier drugs. . .

Possess is usually a pompous way of saying *have*: here the later cephalosporins *have advantages over* the earlier ones (estate agents deal in desirable properties).

PREDICATED/based on, depend on, underlie

To predicate means *to affirm*. The use of *predicated on* for *based on* is American. *Based on* and *depends on* are not the same: an outcome is based on a rule but depends on a condition.

> The interpretation of these data is clearly predicated on the completeness of case ascertainment.

How the data are interpreted *depends on*, but is not *based on*, how completely the cases are ascertained. Put more simply: *Interpretation of the data depends on the accuracy of diagnosis.*

Predicate does not mean *underlie*, which turns the meaning of the word around and suggests the outcome determines the rule or condition:

> [To see whether] there is an overall aetiology for [deviant sexuality we must] look at the forces which predicate all sexuality.

The writer meant forces underlying sexuality, not forces based on or depending on sexuality; nor that the forces affirm sexuality (see also AETIOLOGY).

PREFERENTIAL/preferable

> . . .it would seem preferential to omit percutaneous sutures. . .

A patient who is treated sooner than others is receiving preferential treatment. A treatment that is clinically better than other treatments is the preferable treatment. Preferential treatment is not necessarily preferable treatment.

***PRIOR TO/before*

> The skin was prepared prior to venepuncture. . .

> Spirometry was performed prior to treatment with nebulised salbutamol.

Prior to is preferred to *before* by most medical writers (see p. 89). There are grammatical reasons why *prior to* is incorrect but a better reason for writing *before* is that '*before* is simpler, better known and more natural, and therefore preferable' (Gowers). Bryson is less forgiving and describes *prior to* as 'longer, clumsier and awash with pretension'. Trask writes, 'This ghastly thing has recently become almost a disease'.

Prior to is more tolerable when much more than just the temporal sense of *before* is implied, which is not often so in medical writing. *Prior* is an adjective similar in meaning to *previous* but with connotations of being more important: compare *he had a prior appointment* with *he had a previous appointment*.

PROTOCOL/programme

Protocol, to mean the order in which things were planned or in which things were done during a clinical trial, is American usage (*COD*): 'a record of experimental observations etc.'. The meanings of protocol in English usage are: draft of diplomatic document; formal statement of transaction; observation of official formality or etiquette.

Nonetheless protocol is a useful word, although some may disagree. The possible alternatives are *programme* (*COD*: descriptive notice of series of events), which risks confusion with computer program; or *scheme* (see REGIME, below), which does not convey the strict, ordered, conduct of scientific study.

QUANTITATE/QUANTIFY, *count, measure*

Prefer *count* and *measure* if that is what you mean.

RAISON D'ÊTRE/RATIONALE *reason*

Success and absence of complications with one patient should not become the raison d'être for treating all patients similarly.

Beware of using foreign phrases unless you know their exact meaning (see p. 191). *Raison d'être* does not mean *reason*, the word needed here. It means its exact translation: reason for existence. The variation of disease in time and place is the *raison d'être* for epidemiology.

As less than one half of sore throats is likely to be caused by sensitive bacteria, it is important to have a personal rationale for prescribing them.

Medical treatments rely on more than personal whim, even though *rationale* suggests a more formal assessment than *reason*. There are other faults here. *Less* should be *fewer* (p. 70), and sore throats needs the plural *are* (p. 146). The pronoun *them* refers to antibiotics in a previous sentence. The danger in not repeating *antibiotics* is misconnection to the wrong antecedent noun (p. 171).

Try: *As fewer than half of all sore throats are likely to be caused by sensitive bacteria, it is important to have clear reasons for prescribing antibiotics.*

We prefer *half of* to *50% of* (see p. 95), but *all* is then needed before *sore throats*. An alternative is *half the sore throats*.

**REGIME*/prescription, scheme, regimen*

A Transfusion Regime

These authors proposed a simple regimen using a continuous intravenous infusion of an insulin–glucose–potassium solution. . .

Regime (*COD*): a method of government; the conditions under which a scientific process occurs. Why use this word when we have *prescription* (*COD*): a physician's direction for the composition and use of medicine? Other possible words are *treatment* or *regimen* – although this last is best used to imply a change in the way of life, for instance a beta-adrenergic blocker with a low-salt diet and exercise.

There is a good, simple word, which is correct for both examples, *scheme* (*COD*): a systematic arrangement proposed or in operation; a plan of action.

REGULAR/normal, usual

[These drugs] are regularly examined using techniques. . .

Regular can mean (*COD*) uniformly or calculably in time. Here the writer was referring to the techniques used *normally*, that is the currently standard techniques, before going on to describe a new one. *Regular* for *normal* is American usage.

Clinicians rarely examine drugs, that is usually the job of the chemists or pharmacologists; clinicians examine the effects of the drugs. *Investigate*, *study* or *describe* might be a better word, depending on the context.

RELATION/RELATIONSHIP/CORRELATION

. . .which describes the relation between the original tumour and the site of recurrence.

The relation between the size of infarct and the increase in serum enzymes. . .

A *relation* (*COD*) is what one person or thing has to do with another. Both these examples are correct, but *correlation* (*COD*: mutual relation between two things) is a better word for the second.

> . . .an intimate relationship between the laryngoscope blade and the hyoid bone.

Some authorities hold that one can only have a *relation* between people, and that relations are aunts and uncles. The definition in the *COD* is clearly wider than that. *Relationships*, particularly if intimate, are best left to consenting adults; the example is an absurd way to write that *the laryngoscope blade must be close to the hyoid bone*, which gives the required sense of (*COD*) only a short distance from. (See ASSOCIATED WITH.)

> An interactive relationship exists between the learner and the learning environment.

The word *student*, as applied to anyone who is being taught, is somehow held these days to be too suggestive of young people, or perhaps of troublesome people who experiment with drugs. The awful word *learner* has replaced it. This short sentence also includes *relationship*, *EXISTS* and *ENVIRONMENT*. The sentence means *It matters where you teach*.

REPRESENTS/is

> Tissue expansion represents an important new approach to. . .

Unless one is considering one of a class of similar treatments, *represents* is a pompous way of writing *is*.

> Further work on the course of this disease represents a high-priority need.

Here *represents* fulfils its secret role as a good indicator of poor style; changing it to *is* doesn't do enough because the sentence is topsy-turvy. *There is great need of further work on (understanding) the course of this disease*. (*Priority* is a word much in favour with those trying to distribute health resources fairly. It has spawned (see p. 69) *prioritize* and *prioritization*, words that are ugly and difficult to pronounce. When spoken, *prioritization* is easily misheard as *privatization*.)

> It is currently believed that the electrical activity [of the electroencephalogram] represents the collective post-synaptic potential activity. . .

The electroencephalogram is not the collective post-synaptic activity, so *represents* cannot be replaced by *is*. But *represents* is not correct either because the electroencephalogram cannot *stand in place of* that activity. Better is *reflects* or *is due to* (see DUE TO). *Currently* is superfluous (and better not used in a description of electricity).

RESPIRATORY/VENTILATORY

Some believe that *respiration* should be reserved to describe cellular events, the utilization of oxygen and production of carbon dioxide in the tissues, and *ventilation* to describe the movement of gases in and out of the lungs. Others define *respiration* as the physiology of events occurring between the air and the tissues; *ventilation* is therefore a part of respiration, but *respiration* is not a part of ventilation. Thus the response to inhaled carbon dioxide can be described either as the *ventilatory* response or as the *respiratory* response – but one must be consistent: choose one or other term and use it throughout the text.

The best word to use is often *breathing*, a word of Anglo-Saxon origin.

RESULTS/FINDINGS

These words are used interchangeably to mean the measured outcome of a study. If the work is purely descriptive and there has not been any attempt to investigate the effects of an external influence on the system under study, then *findings* may be the better word (see DATA, p. 148).

**REVEAL/SHOW

Reveal has connotations of revelation, magic and the sudden whipping aside of curtains. Prefer the simpler *show*. *Exhibit* and *manifest* are similar words to avoid (see also DEMONSTRATE).

ROLE/part

Prostaglandins play a major role in inflammation.

Roles played and parts played have almost identical meanings but, if these phrases must be used in medical writing, at least *play a part* has the merit of being the correct idiom and euphonious. (See also Metaphor, p. 156.)

SACRIFICE/KILL

. . .and blood was taken for analysis prior to sacrifice of the animal.

A *sacrifice* is a religious rite or (*COD*) the giving up of a valued thing for the sake of another that is more worthy or more important or more urgent. Do not use *sacrifice* when you mean *kill*. A similar debasement is likely to happen to *assassinate* if the media persist in applying it to when gangsters and terrorists are murdered.

    The incorrect use here of PRIOR TO for *before* has caused an ambiguity: the blood was taken before death, but the example reads as if the analysis was done before death. It should read . . .*and blood for later analysis was taken before the animal was killed.*

SERVES/is

The first. . .serves as a reminder that. . .

Is will do; *serves* adds nothing to the sense. *The first reminds us.* . . is better.

These cases serve to emphasize. . .

Omit. *Serve to emphasize* means *emphasize.*

SHOW/have

The mitochondria showed fewer cristae.

Showed is only a minor inflation when compared with EXHIBIT in this context (and one meaning of *show* is *to manifest* (*COD*)), but what is wrong with *had*?

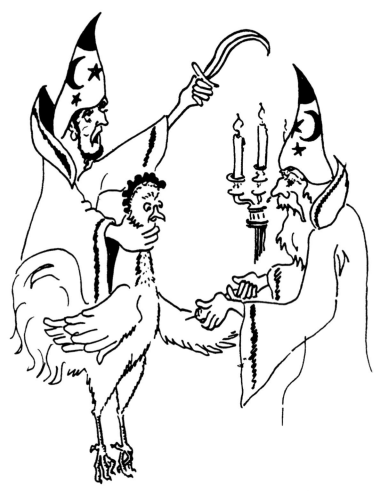

. . .blood was taken for analysis prior to the sacrifice of the animal.

SIMPLISTIC/simple

A simplistic explanation for these observations is that. . .

Simplistic means oversimplified or affectedly naive. To describe a colleague's or rival's explanation as simplistic might be taken as an insult if they know the proper meaning of the word.

SPECIALITY/specialty

Choux pastry, tripe and onions and Sauerkraut are regional specialities; radiology, pathology and surgery are medical specialties. Americans use only the one word *specialty* for both these meanings.

SPECTRUM/RANGE

> . . .few reports of its use in paediatric practice with its different spectrum of pathology.

Spectrum refers to wavelengths of electromagnetic radiation. The *COD* lists spectrum as (figuratively) the entire range of anything arranged by degree, quality, etc. The sense here is simply *range*.

Despite this, the phrase *broad-spectrum antibiotics* is in common usage.

Pathology (see p. 76) should not be used, as it was in this example, as a synonym for *disease*.

SYNERGY/COOPERATION

Synergy means two factors having a combined effect greater than the sum of their separate effects, in other words, more than just additive. Do not write synergy as a synonym for *cooperation*, or *working together*, unless synergy is really what will result. Managers and politicians are fond of synergy, which some may interpret as obstruction.

SUPERIOR TO/better than

Superior and *inferior* are anatomical terms meaning *above and below with respect to the standing human body*. If writing that one method or drug is preferred to another write *better than*. (The expansion *the superiority of* is even worse than *superior to*.) *Inferior to* is not so easily replaced, but *not as good as* conveys the sense. *Worse than* is usually used as a comparison of two things both of which are not good.

TARGET/aim, objective

Target, like *focus*, is fashionable and liked particularly by politicians and administrators, presumably because it sounds more solid than the preferable *aim* or *objective*.

Target is used increasingly as a verb but this use should be avoided.

> It is necessary for us to know who operates on children so that we can target our activities [a questionnaire] accurately.

This is typical 'adminspeak' for *We need to know who operates on children so that we can question the right people.* Those who receive the questionnaire are the *intended* recipients not the *target* recipients.

TECHNOLOGY/technique

Technology has come to mean more than just the science of the practical arts so if your lab switches to using, say, gene probes you can write that you are involved in a 'new technology'. But a new way of doing a particular thing, be it a lab test or a surgical operation, is at best a 'new technique' not a technology. It is also, simply, a new *method* (see p. 75).

An American speaking of a new test for HIV said that 'the whole technology takes place in the test-tube'. They must have large test-tubes in America.

USING/with, by

> Samples were analysed using a mass spectrometer. . .

Using *using* where an appropriate preposition will suffice is one of the easiest and most common ways of introducing unnecessary complication into a sentence. It also offers the temptation to invert the sentence and write a 'dangling participle' (see p. 184). *Samples were analysed with a mass spectrometer* or *by mass spectrometry* are the better alternatives.

***UTILIZE, UTILIZATION/use (verb or noun)*

Do not write *utilize* simply as a synonym of *use* (see EMPLOY). Valid contexts for *utilization* in medicine would be utilization of foods as sources of energy, of substrates in metabolic pathways, or of resources in managing a service.

The following examples are not of simple substitution for *use*, they are indicators of generally lazy writing.

> . . .all studies of portal vein perfusion have utilised the obliterated umbilical veins for cannulation.

It was the investigators, not the studies, that did the using. Invert the sentence: . . .*the obliterated umbilical veins were cannulated in all studies.*

Utilisation of an implantable reservoir may allow a more prolonged use of. . .

There would be little point in implanting a reservoir but not using it. *An implantable reservoir may allow. . .* is better. Other similar unneeded phrases are BY MEANS OF, BY THE PRESENCE OF, AND BY THE USE OF.

. . .by fully utilizing their. . .

Better as . . .*by making full use of their. . ..*

VARIATION/VARIABILITY

None of the differences were statistically significant due to marked variation. . .

The writers were measuring the concentration of a drug in sequential samples of plasma. *Variation* then refers to differences in concentration with time in one particular patient, and *variability* to the differences in concentration between patients at particular sampling times. *Variability* is the correct word here.

The example contains other errors. NONE requires the singular *was* (see p. 146); and DUE TO is used incorrectly as an adverb. Another error is the writers' assumption that the variability prevented the results being statistically significant (see p. 131).

Some referees and journals hold that application of the word *significant* implies a *statistical* judgement. Under these circumstances, *statistically* should be omitted. (*Important* is often a better word than *significant*.)

VIEWPOINT/view, point

. . .a similar viewpoint was expressed by. . .

A viewpoint is taken; a view is expressed; a point is made.

VIRTUALLY/almost

Almost is the older word in English by at least 600 years, and has one syllable less. The increasing use of virtual in expressions such as *virtual reality*, which is not reality at all, is another reason for preferring *almost*. One of us spotted this at an outdoor event:

> This is a real simulator.

So much for reality.

**VISUALIZE/see*

To visualize is to make visible to the eye – *usually the mind's eye*; one can visualize without seeing. It is reasonable to write visualize when referring to techniques that produce images only on a film or a television screen; acceptable, perhaps, when using fibre-optic instruments. Otherwise use *see*; visualize should not be debased and devalued by indiscriminate use or incorrect usage.

> . . .on laryngoscopy the vocal cords could not be visualized. . .

Seen is better. And . . .*only the posterior ends of the cords were visible* or *could be seen* is better than the less explanatory statement *could not be fully visualized*.

> Aspiration of liquid mercury is usually benign, although roentgenologic visualization of mercury globules may be evident for many years.

To write of visualization by X-ray is acceptable, though . . .*roentgenologic* [*X-ray* in UK English] *evidence remains for many years* is neater.

-WISE

There is a tendency that started in America to tack *-wise* to the ends of words: *Rhythm-wise, the electrocardiogram was normal*. This is an ugly way of saying or writing: *The electrocardiogram showed normal rhythm*. In statistics, '*pair-wise* comparisons' is probably respectable.

5
Superfluous words

Some common examples

Scientific writing in general, and medical writing in particular, is muddied by superfluous words. These masquerade as part of convention but are actually just catch-phrases or padding: the literary equivalent of clearing the throat. We select as common culprits *basis, case, conditions, essentially, feature, function, grounds, instance, nature, situation, type, very.* These sorts of word usually add nothing; they are words for words' sake. When you can recognize them as such, delete them and restructure the sentence.

BASIS

The patients were examined on a daily basis means that patients were examined *daily.*

Samples of blood were taken on a regular basis means that samples were taken *regularly.*

These adverbial phrases (*on a daily basis, on a regular basis*) can usually be replaced by the simple adverbs (*daily, regularly*).

> It should be possible to perform 25% of all operations on a day case basis by the year. . .

There is no adverb *day-casely,* but why not *as day cases?* (And incidentally why not *a quarter* for '25%'?)

A *one-to-one basis* is a fashionable phrase; it means individual(ly).

BASICALLY, see ESSENTIALLY

CASE

Searching for *case* is worthwhile; it can almost always be replaced or deleted (see p. 126). It is correct usage in *We report 13 cases of diabetes* or *Atropine should be available in case a bradycardia occurs,* although *Atropine should be available to correct any bradycardia* is better.

> It is too early to judge if this is the case or not.

Replace *the case or not* with *so.* To be grammatically correct, the second half of the example should be in the *subjunctive* and should read *if this be so.* The subjunctive is a *mood* of verb that we all use (when we tell someone, 'Be quiet!' or advise them, 'If I were you. . .') but it is rarely recognized for what it is and is used less now than formerly.

CONDITIONS

> Anaesthesia under civil war conditions.

Civil war conditions are conditions simulating those of a civil war. The writer was describing a particular civil war, for which *Anaesthesia during a civil war* is correct.

Conditions can be a useful word if a set of circumstances has been described (bad weather, under fire, a lack of drugs and unskilled personnel) to which you later wish to refer: *Under these conditions it is important to think clearly.*

EPIDEMIC

Epidemic is favoured by pressure groups. It has been given overtones of culpability. Authors write of an epidemic of breast cancer, as if there is a conspiracy to harm women, or of an epidemic of asthma, blaming the pollutant by-products of the capitalist–industrial complex (although they still drive their children to school in their gas-guzzling cars). Breast cancer or asthma could be epidemic, but they are not: the defining feature of an epidemic is the widespread occurrence of a disease at a particular time – and strictly the disease should be infectious. Metaphorical use allows epidemic to apply to any 'sudden, widespread occurrence of an undesirable phenomenon' (*COD*), for example (to reactionary commentators) the wearing of baseball caps backwards. Just because a disease is becoming more prevalent, for example asthma, does not make it an epidemic, although the rate at which Western populations are putting on weight probably justifies talk of an epidemic of obesity.

Avoid *epidemic proportions*. A sense of proportion is needed: when everything is an epidemic, nothing is.

ESSENTIALLY

The abdominal pain is essentially colicky across the lower abdomen. . .

The adjectives *basic, essential* and *fundamental* have retained clearer meanings than the adverbs formed from them. These adverbs, *basically, essentially* and *fundamentally* are much used in speech as padding to give speakers time to think. Writers have had time to think and should not use padding. Try not to use these words at all; either delete them or replace them with explicit words or phrases that give your intended meaning. *Mainly* or *most commonly* would be better in the example, but does *colicky* need qualification at all?

The pain is described *across the lower abdomen*, so *abdominal* is redundant. This leaves *There is colicky lower abdominal pain. . ..*

> **This weighting, however, does not correspond to any actual preference of the respondent: it is basically an artefact, generated by the requirement for consistency between questions that address different issues. . ..**

Basically weakens the statement that follows the colon, which needs the bold 'it is an artefact. . ..'. *Between questions on different topics* is better than 'questions that address different issues. . ..'.

FEATURE

Hypogonadism is a recognized feature of chronic renal failure and chronic liver disease.

Do not use this construction, or the similar *has been described in*, ambiguously to imply that the symptom or sign is known but rare; if that is what you mean, be more explicit (see p. 116).

A *feature* is a recognized sign: the word *recognized* is unnecessary. Either *Hypogonadism occurs in* or *Hypogonadism is a feature of* is better here.

If the list is just of symptoms, then one should be specific: *Symptoms of chronic renal failure include lethargy, headache, nausea. . ..* If the list includes symptoms and signs from many systems then valid usage would be: *Features of chronic renal failure include lethargy, acidosis, hyperkalaemia, bone cysts. . ..*

FUNCTION

> . . .below-knee amputation is preferable to above-knee amputation in regard to function. . .

The whole phrase *in regard to function* should be deleted, and the specific function of the knee joint (mobility, stability) should be defined: *. . . below-knee amputation preserves mobility better than above-knee. . ..*

> . . .the Bain circuit has been shown to be identical to the classic T-piece in terms of its function.

Here, *function* is a pointer to the generally poor style that includes the unnecessary word *classic* (*COD*: perfectly typical). The example shows well how some writers find it impossible to write anything simply: all they are saying is that *the Bain circuit functions as an ordinary T-piece.*

Function has given birth to *functionality*, a word common in computer manuals. Something with *versatile functionality* is *useful.*

> When the impact of an electronic medical records system is investigated, we suggest that its actual use should be considered rather than its claimed functionality.

We will allow the authors the ironic use of functionality here, as we have no doubt that functionality is what was used in attempts to sell them the equipment. However, *rather than the manufacturer's claims* is more explicit.

FUNDAMENTALLY, see ESSENTIALLY

GROUNDS

> . . .a heterogeneous group of tumours on epidemiological grounds.

This is *an epidemiologically heterogeneous group of tumours.*

The diagnosis of epididymo-orchitis is made on clinical grounds. . .

The adverb has been expanded (see BASIS). *The diagnosis is made clinically.*

INSTANCE

At reoperation, abscesses were found in the pancreatic bed in all instances.

The abscesses were not found in instances, they were found in patients.

NATURE

. . .symptoms of a neurological nature. . .

Symptoms of a neurological nature are *neurological symptoms.*

. . .may forewarn of events of a more serious nature. . .

Better as *forewarn of more serious events.*

The serious nature of air accidents occurring during infusion. . .

Better as *The seriousness of. . ..* The 'air accidents' that the writers were describing were air emboli.

The hyperosmolar nature of the contrast medium may induce pulmonary oedema.

Hyperosmolar nature is *hyperosmolarity. Induce* is not wrong, but *cause* is better.

PROCESS

The word *process* has intruded hugely into medical writing. Any value the intrusion may have had is probably now debased. The origin of *process* could be in the philosophical attitude of, for example, social sciences, which seeks to emphasize 'states of being in process' to contrast to distinct and absolute definitions. In medicine, process can be added to anything, but usually adds nothing. The commonly seen *disease process* instead of just *disease* might charitably be seen as a reminder that diseases are not fixed or absolute conditions, but even the simplest level of medical education conveys this point without the need for quasi-tautological phrases such as *cancer process* and *inflammatory process*.

> This study helps to provide an understanding of the factors influencing the decision making process in people with symptoms of a heart attack.

Process is especially common in the phrase *decision making process*: *This study helps us to understand how decisions are made. . ..*

> Asphyxia is a low-frequency event in the birthing process in developed countries.

This means no more than *Asphyxia during birth is uncommon. . ..*

> The ageing process can make people increasingly vulnerable through erosion of their coping abilities. . .

The ageing process is no different from ageing. *As people age, they are more vulnerable because they cope less well.* (See also Nouns as adjectives (p. 162).)

A similar word is *experience*:

> The aim of the MB ChB programme is to provide a learning experience which produces doctors who are capable of addressing the perceived health needs of the nation. . .

Perhaps the programme (why not a course?) is based on the same philosophy as the hotel promising that 'A dining experience is enhanced when the harmony of food and wine synergy is in concert with the service.'

SITUATION/SITUATED

Situation has become so misused in the last few years that it is probably best not to use it even when it would be correct. Television sport commentators must take a lot of blame ('And Cambridge are in a sinking situation!'), but doctors are picking up the habit: *in the intensive care situation* means nothing more nor less than *in the intensive care unit*; *in an emergency situation* means *in an emergency*.

Situation is correct in *The situation of the intensive care unit is important*, although *the siting* is better if referring to the position of the unit relative to other wards.

The lower oesophageal sphincter is a physiological sphincter, situated at the lower end of the oesophagus, which. . .

Omit *situated*.

. . .situated in the immediate vicinity of. . .

Few are suitably situated in relation to the operating theatre.

These two examples are from the same paper. *Situated* can be omitted from the first – but the whole phrase can be replaced by *next to*. The second contains also the *indicator* (see p. 118) IN RELATION TO; and *suitably situated in relation to* means *close enough to*.

TYPE

. . .trolleys should be of the tipping type. . .

Strictly, it should be *trolleys should be capable of being tipped* because trolleys do not themselves tip; people tip them. The phrase *a tipping trolley* is well understood, though, and *trolleys should tip* is less cumbersome.

VERY

Gowers advises that it is wise to be sparing of *very*. There is no such thing as 'scientific English' but *very* is an unscientific word. Avoid it.

Unnecessary adverbs

ABOLISH, ELIMINATE, FATAL, PREVENT, VITAL

These words should be modified with caution. *Absolutely vital* is incorrect because *vital* means *necessary to life* and needs no further emphasis. The same considerations apply to the other words.

The response is totally abolished in Group 1 patients by. . .

. . .any leak across the piston is entirely eliminated.

Abolish, eliminate and *prevent* should not be modified by adverbs of degree because the verbs imply totality and there cannot be partial abolition or partial elimination. If a response is not abolished, or a leak not eliminated, then one should use reduced or decreased.

It is correct to write *sometimes abolished* or *usually eliminated* (adverbs of frequency) if, to use the examples above, the response was abolished in some patients but not in others, or the leak was eliminated on some occasions.

> They found that haemorrhage into a pancreatic abscess was uniformly fatal.

Again, *fatal* can be modified by adverbs of frequency, but only with care by adverbs of degree. It is reasonable to write *rarely fatal, sometimes fatal* or *usually fatal*. The simple statement that haemorrhage was fatal implies without need of modification that all affected patients died. If you want to stress the outcome, then *always fatal* is better than uniformly fatal as *uniformly* implies that the route to, not just the cause, of death was identical in all patients.

Repetition

Do not write the same thing twice. There is no easy way to spot this error of style with a word processor. Reading through the text, asking all the time, 'Is this word or phrase really necessary?', can help to spot tautologies.

> The results are plotted graphically. . .

Omit *graphically*. *Plotting* implies the drawing of a graph. Writers sometimes write *represented graphically*, which is a circumlocutory way of saying *plotted*.

> This arrangement avoids the rebreathing of previously exhaled gases from the expiratory limb. . .

The definition of rebreathing is the inspiring of expired air hence *This arrangement avoids rebreathing* is sufficient. *To avoid* means *to bypass*, and the sense here is not *avoidance* but *prevention*: *This prevents rebreathing* is correct.

> . . .fully complies with the requirements needed in [current testing of lung function]. . .

Write either *requirements of* or *needs of*. (In the original example, *current testing of lung function* was written as 'modern pulmonalogical examinations'!)

> . . .operations of varying magnitude, ranging from simple drainage to a full laparotomy.

The extent of operation is expressed three times in this example: *of varying magnitude, ranging,* and *from. . .to*: *operations from simple drainage to full laparotomy* is sufficient.

> Timing of removal varied from between 10 and 16 days. . .

The repetition (the use of *varied from* and *between*) has caused a grammatical error: one says *between 10 and 16*, but *from 10 to 16* (see also pp. 121 and 124).

> It is possible that our results might have been better had we. . .

> In some instances the possibility exists that the solvent, and not the drug, may be responsible for adverse reactions.

It is sometimes wise not to be dogmatic, but do not hedge to an unnecessary degree.[17] *It is possible that* can be omitted from the first example. *Sometimes* can replace the construction *In some instances the possibility exists that* in the second.

> . . .failure to intubate can potentially lead to fatality.

Although this is improved by omitting *potentially*, it is better to make the clear statement *failure to intubate can cause death*. The dramatic *failure to intubate can kill* may be taken to indicate intent and is better avoided in formal writing (see FATALITY).

> Myoclonus and myelinolysis may follow as sequelae.

A sequel necessarily follows: *Myoclonus and myelinolysis may be sequelae.*

6

Imprecise words and phrases

Some words are used as 'catch-alls', when a little thought would suggest a better word. Sometimes *associate, involve, concern* and *regard* are appropriate; but often they indicate laziness.

Lavoisier believed it impossible to dissociate language from science or science from language.[10] Sloppy language means sloppy science.

If you find the following words in your first draft, think carefully about whether they could be replaced by more precise ones.

ACHIEVE, ATTAIN

If *achieve* cannot be replaced by *obtain* or *reach*, then it might indicate that the construction of the sentence should be altered. *Achieve* is commonly superfluous.

> Maximum pressures are said to be attained after. . .

Attain, achieve and *reach* can all mean *to get there*, but *reach* means just that; it is a good simple word that does not colour its surroundings. A guide to the best verb can be the noun formed from it: the achievement of a lifetime's ambition; the attainment of a great, perhaps metaphorical, height. Looked at in this way, these words are not good ones for our rather more mundane purpose. *Maximum pressures are said to be attained after*. . . is rather grand for a scientific report. The best verb here, though, is *occur: are said to occur after*. . . (even though *occur* is suffering from overuse (p. 40)).

> The only way in which a lower rate can be achieved . . .

The writers were discussing the settings on a ventilator: *obtain* is perfectly good. Changing from the passive *to be achieved* to the active *to obtain* makes the example less clumsy: *The only way to obtain a lower rate. . ..* (See Use of the passive voice, pp. 139–143.)

Even *obtain* can be replaced with a shorter word – *get*, an inelegant word. It is not good style to develop an obsession for short words any more than it is to write only long words. Some long words can be replaced only by a long string of monosyllabic words; the longer word may then be better style. Better still in the last example is *The only way to decrease the rate. . . .*

> However, in only *x*% of limbs was success achieved by this method . . .

This is correct usage, one achieves success; but to write simply *However, this method was successful in only x%* . . . is more direct.

> This [reduction of waiting lists] has been achieved by. . .

The correct word is *managed* and suggests that the writer can think clearly.

ADDRESS

The ubiquitous use of *address* to replace just about any verb has so far escaped comment in most style manuals. Perhaps this usage is recent; we cannot believe that Fowler would have overlooked such an overused word. There is almost nothing that cannot be addressed (*COD*: think about and begin to deal with): issues, arguments, definitions, expectations, gaps, inequalities, representativeness, risks, shortages, threats, variations, and even what is right and what is wrong–all have been addressed.

But when arguments are addressed, are they defined, considered, accepted or countered? Are expectations being described, denied or realized? Are variations being analysed, categorized or reduced? The most popular targets for addressing are issues and questions, which is an even higher level of vagueness because the issue or question will be one of definitions, expectations, gaps, inequalities and so on. If a question is addressed, is it framed, asked or answered?

Any verb that can be used to mean both 'to question' and 'to answer' is a word to be wary of.

Only two things can be addressed: envelopes and audiences. All questions are posed; some questions are answered. Other addressing is waffle, risking the inference of an action that may not be intended.

> Clinical governance ... will also be seen as a way of addressing concerns about the quality of health care.

> Quality improvement must address the whole range of performances.

> ... the tenacity with which the problem is addressed is very important to the standing of the NHS and the healthcare professions in the eyes of the public.

These three examples are from the same much-quoted article about clinical governance. We don't want clinical governance to address concerns, the range and the problem; we want it to answer concerns, cover the range and solve the problem. Address is the perfect verb for those unprepared to find the right word; avoid it.

> An editorial addressing these articles provides insight into the similarities and differences in the trials and discusses the problems that must be addressed if [this] is to be a major therapeutic advance.

Address twice in the same sentence, meaning *prompted by* the first time and *solved* the second. The new therapy will not be an advance if the problems are only thought about; they will need to be solved.

There is something else that can properly be addressed, a golf ball, but neither of us is qualified to offer advice.

ASSOCIATED WITH

Ischaemic heart disease and peripheral vascular disease are associated; they tend to occur together. They may *have the same causation,* but neither causes the other. The association is two-way; one can just as easily write that peripheral vascular disease and ischaemic heart disease are associated.

By comparison, it is unhelpful to write that hypercapnia (an increased partial pressure of carbon dioxide in arterial blood) is associated with hyperventilation when plainly hypercapnia either *causes* hyperventilation (when rebreathing) or *is a result of* blunted ventilatory drive (in chronic obstructive airways disease).

It is extremely important that doctors have a clear idea of the difference between association and causation. Yet there are many papers in the journals in which the distinction is blurred. Case reports are particularly likely to give rise to the erroneous belief that, because B happened after A, A was therefore responsible for B. Commonly, it is not the writers that make the assertion, but the readers who make the assumption. A case report appears; the writers describe B happening after A – it might be Brown *et al.* describing two cases of photophobia in patients with cardiac pacemakers. Before long, further papers appear that have in the Introduction, 'Cardiac pacemakers cause photophobia (Brown *et al.*, 1991). This present study was designed to investigate the effect of two different types of sunglasses on the incidence of this complication. . . .'

The correct sense of *association* is illustrated well by these two examples.

> Fractures of the maxilla and mandible are often associated with a primary head injury and fractures of the cervical spine.

> The association between infection of the lower genital tract by human papillomavirus and intraepithelial neoplasia has been recognised for some time, and an increasing body of evidence suggests that this association is causal rather than casual.

If the association is definitely causal, then use *cause*. Do not use *associate* to imply that a causation is rare.

> The commonest cause of air embolism has been associated with accidental disconnection or misconnection of the junctions . . .

The commonest cause *is* accidental disconnection. The sentence would be better still if reversed: *Misconnection or accidental disconnection of junctions is the commonest cause. . . .*

> Suxamethonium administration is frequently associated with increases in serum potassium and myoglobin.

Write *frequently causes* or, better, *commonly causes*. As drugs do nothing unless given to a patient, the sentence can be shortened: *Suxamethonium commonly causes. . . .*

> The treatment of a pharyngeal pouch by excision has always been associated with a high complication rate . . .

Why not *excision of a pharyngeal pouch causes many complications*?

> The use of regional analgesia may be associated with greater heat loss. . .

Use of regional analgesia may *cause* greater heat loss.

> Autonomic neuropathy is associated with increasing age . . .

This is correct if what is meant is *as patients age they are more likely to have autonomic neuropathy*. It is *not* correct if what is meant is *autonomic neuropathy is more common in the elderly than it is in the young*, which was the context here.

> Ten ml was associated with less cervical blockade.
>
> The larger volume was associated with hoarseness . . .
>
> Larger volumes are associated with an increased incidence of side effects.

These three examples are from the same paper. In the first, *caused* is better. (The full form of 'Ten ml', discussed further on p. 192, is *Ten millilitres*. Some would prefer this to be followed by the plural *were*, not *was*. The alternative view is that the ten millilitres are a unitary dose and *was* is correct.)

In the second example, *caused* is better if the larger volume always caused hoarseness or if the sentence concludes by stating the incidence (*in half the cases*). Otherwise *tended to cause* would be correct.

In the third the sense is *cause* but rephrasing gives *increase the incidence of*. . . .

> . . . and eliminates the risks associated with the increases in lung volume.

Here *associated with* can be omitted: . . . *the risks of increased lung volume*.

> Needle electrodes have been associated with infection, broken needles, and intraneural placement.
>
> During the first 23 months it was noted that stomach cancer was very rarely associated with liver metastases.

Associated with in these examples cannot be replaced by single words. Try: *Needle electrodes may break, cause infection, or damage the nerves* and: *In the first 23 months, few of the patients with stomach cancer had liver metastases*. . . .

You can often decide if *associated* is correct by reversing the order of the associated items; if correct, the sense should remain the same. For instance, the Conservative party is associated with the colour blue; blue is associated with the Conservatives. The second example above implies that, in a series of patients with stomach cancer, few had liver metastases. Reversing the sentence, *Liver metastases were rarely associated with stomach cancer*, implies that, of a series of patients with liver metastases, few had stomach cancer.

Stomach cancer and *liver metastases* are well-established phrases in which nouns are used as adjectives (see p. 162), although many stylists would prefer *cancer of the stomach* and *metastases in the liver.*

> Such operations could theoretically have been associated with sacral plexus damage, causing or contributing to constipation.

This is a clumsy way of writing *Damage to the sacral plexus during these operations could cause or worsen constipation. Contributing* is a poor choice of word. People contribute money to a charity and authors contribute chapters to a book, which is not the sense here.

Writers probably use *associate with* partly because they are wary of ascribing causation without good evidence. It is difficult to see in the last example how anything other than the operation could have caused the damage to the plexus – whether by scalpel, retractor, or other instrument.

> A loop colostomy has been generally preferred to a loop ileostomy because of the problems associated with stoma care in the latter . . .

This needs rewriting (see LATTER, p. 136). *Loop colostomies are generally preferred to loop ileostomies because it is easier to care for an ileal stoma.*

> Tumours greater than 10 cm in diameter were associated with a particularly poor prognosis.

The tumours were the direct cause of the poor prognosis, but replacing *were associated with* by *had* or *caused* is not correct. The original ignores the patients who have the tumours: *Patients with tumours greater than 10 cm in diameter had a particularly poor prognosis.*

A correct use of association is in discussing a numerical index of disease that is linked with outcome. Examples are the neonatal Apgar score, the Glasgow Coma Score, and the intensive care APACHE score. This brings out the connection between *association* and *statistical correlation*. The index can be used as a pointer but is not an exact measure of outcome for an individual.

CONCERN/REGARD

Use *concern* if there is some anxiety; use *regard* to indicate an impression of. For instance: *We were concerned about the study; we regarded it as irrelevant.*

> This report concerns our experience with colectomy . . .

Concern can mean *pertain to*, so this usage is correct, but it would be better to write the more direct *This is a report of our experience.*

> The major concern regarding this incision is the higher incidence of dehiscence . . .

The writers may well have been concerned or worried about the higher incidence, but how can this concern regard? *The major problem with this incision* is better. *Main* is better than MAJOR.

> . . . a surgical failure as far as her pain was concerned . . .

The construction *as far as . . . was concerned*, as with much imprecise writing, can be made to apply to anything: the rash was on his face as far as distribution was concerned; he was 1.73 metres as far as height was concerned. Be precise and direct: *surgery failed to relieve her pain*. A feature of imprecise writing is that sections taken out of context often make no sense: *her pain was concerned* is meaningless.

> Accidents most often concerned young children or the elderly.

The accidents should have been the concern of everyone; the young children and – not *or* – the elderly were *involved* (see below). Even then it is an unsatisfactory way of writing *Young children and the elderly* (or *elderly people*) *had the most accidents.*

> The individual choice of the patient concerning therapy is confronted with the perception of therapeutic needs by the treating doctor.

This may mean *Patients choosing a particular treatment will be influenced by their doctor*, or (this really *is* an obscure sentence), *The patient's choice of treatment may conflict with that of the doctor.*

DETERMINE

A reviewer of the second edition of the book chided us for missing 'the umbrella word of all time': determine. Once drawn to our attention, it was unmissable. *Determine* in the sense (COD) 'be a decisive factor in regard to' is a proper use:

> . . . non-diabetic dizygotic and monozygotic twin siblings of patients with type 1 diabetes had a similar high prevalence of islet cell autoantibody

expression, suggesting that islet cell autoimmunity is mainly environmentally determined.

Otherwise, *determine* is usually better replaced by a more precise word.

This study was undertaken to determine which method is the better approximation.

Suitable replacements are ascertain and decide.

The area of each projection was determined using the DispImage computer program.

Measured or estimated is better.

Prognosis is determined mainly by the degree of left ventricular dysfunction and the extent of residual jeopardised myocardium,

Prognosis depends on the degree is better.

ENVIRONMENT

This word is creeping into use when *surroundings, conditions* or some similar word would be better. *Environment* is (*COD*) surrounding objects, region or conditions, especially circumstances of life of person or society. It is a poor word for describing reduced gastric acidity ('This study aimed to provide a safer gastric environment') or the difference between the front and back seats of a car ('The rear seat environment is different from that of the front').

In recent years, we have come under pressure to raise the levels of patient services we provide, usually in an environment of resource constraint.

CONDITIONS is better than *environment*. The sentence means that *we have been pushed to give more and more for less and less*.

HIGHLIGHT/assess, confirm, describe, emphasize, stress, underline

The report highlighted the costs to the NHS . . . of admissions . . .

. . . the survey . . . highlighted the need for systematic evaluation of caesarean section.

Highlight is defined in the *COD* as to bring into prominence or to draw attention to. Highlight occurs too often in Discussions: *This study highlights the importance of good nutrition.* Depending on the sense, *emphasizes, stresses* or *confirms* would be better. Leave highlighting for something done with a fluorescent pen – not least because as an emphatic word it has been played out by politicians, and the media that report their doings.

INVOLVED

Fowler regarded *involve* as an overworked 'general-purpose verb that saves the trouble of precise thought'. Precise thought is precisely what a good scientist should use, and this applies as much to the writing as to the work that it describes.

> The community nursing services are therefore likely to become involved more frequently . . .

Involve implies a degree of complexity – rather more than just need or participation. This is correct usage of involve: the community nursing services encompass the administration, the staff, and the nurses' work.

> Monitoring involved cannulation of the radial artery for the recording of arterial pressure . . .

Monitoring *included* cannulation of the artery, but this still awkward construction (the *cannulation* wasn't monitored; cannulation *enabled* the monitoring) can be avoided by *Arterial pressure was recorded from the cannulated radial artery. . .* (even though the word *monitoring* is correct, see MONITOR).

> High blocks above the T5 dermatome would involve undesirable interruption . . .

High blocks would *cause* interruption.

> The study involved 15 consenting healthy adult males . . .

Fifteen subjects *took part* or *were included* in the study; it was the investigators who were *involved.*

There are two other points of style in this example. First, *adult males,* unless of another species, are *men.* Secondly, the writers clearly lacked any sensibility! Patients who give consent to take part in clinical trials should not be referred to as *consenting adult males* (though consent*ed* may do). Rewritten, the example reads: *Fifteen healthy men gave consent to take part in the study.* . . .

> . . . because of the high gas velocities and rapid changes in flow direction involved.

Involved can be omitted.

> . . . continued uptake is involved in the stabilisation . . .

Implicated is a better single word, but *continued uptake helps to stabilise* is better still. Implication has connotations of intent.

MAJOR

Bryson considers *major* a severely overworked word, which 'brings a kind of tofu quality to much writing, giving it bulk but little additional flavour'. Hardly a programme on television appears that is not *A major new serial* or *A major investigation into* . . ., and medical conferences are now announced in the same way. They usually advertise well-known authorities who will give *keynote lectures* and chair *plenary sessions*. These two expressions are euphemisms for introductory rambles and discussion from the floor, the time left for discussion depending on the extent to which the keynote speakers overrun.

Major is correct in *major operation*. It should not be used instead of a more explicit adjective such as large (or largest), important, serious, obvious or extensive. These last four can be preceded by *most* if appropriate. Often *major* can be replaced by the simple *main*.

> A major goal of the [new] journal will be to report on the developing world.

An important aim of the new journal. . . .

Minor does not cause the same difficulty. Advertising a *minor conference on joint replacement* would probably not attract too many people. *Minor operation, minor complications* and *minor morbidity* are all useful expressions and are not as dismissive of the possible feelings of the patient as substituting *unimportant*. *Illness* may be better than *morbidity* (see p. 63).

Not just single words but also phrases can be imprecise. A common example is to write of the *social implications* of a disease or condition. If you can define the implications more precisely – caring for a family, the effects on a demanding job, approaching examinations – always do so.

TOOL/INSTRUMENT

We are indebted to Jenny Caddy, an anaesthetist from Northern England, for drawing our attention to the way no one is ever happy to talk about what precisely is being used to measure or manipulate, preferring instead to refer to tools or instruments.

> Patients will answer standard, validated questionnaires before and after undergoing surgery. . . These tools give valuable insight into what patients themselves want.

But tools are hammers, chisels, spades; instruments are scalpels, forceps, scissors. Or in another sphere, violins and oboes. Questionnaires are not tools or instruments, although they are a way or method of determining opinions. This common use of tool is metaphorical (see p. 156) and should be avoided.

> Lifelong learning will give NHS staff the tools of knowledge to offer the most modern, effective and high quality care to patients.

What are the tools of knowledge? It is enough to say that lifelong learning (a cliché: see p. 156) enables staff to give better care.

> Opportunities for further clinical trials include the impact of EOA, EGTA, PTL, and ETC on morbidity and mortality for patients resuscitated in the hospital setting. No large series has compared these tools with endotracheal intubation or pre-hospital surgical intervention. Morbidity may be higher with these instruments, since adequate ventilation may not always be assured.

Ignoring the abbreviations, which are four techniques of non-invasive ventilation of the lungs, our main comment is that the writer is so frightened of repetition (*techniques* would have done each time) that the techniques become both tools and instruments. This is bound to cloud thought, because the techniques themselves require equipment, that is, tools and instruments. Writing of the *impact* of something used to compress the chest is also not a good choice of word. The whole passage, the last paragraph of a *Lancet* editorial, is better rewritten: *It would be helpful to know how EOA, EGTA, PTL, and ETC affect outcome in patients resuscitated in hospital, especially as no large study has compared them with endotracheal intubation or pre-hospital surgical intervention. Because ventilation cannot be assured using the non-invasive techniques, they may cause more complications.*

7

Superfluous phrases

There are important differences between writing and speaking. Spoken information needs to be padded, repeated in different ways, given a number of different emphases; all help the audience to follow the speaker's ideas. When reading, readers read at their own pace, stopping and re-reading as they need to (although the need for a lot of re-reading indicates a lack of clarity): the padding is not necessary.

Common superfluities

The following examples of the most common superfluities in medical writing would mostly seem inelegant even in speech. Yet they easily slip past the glazed eyes of the hard-pressed reader as part of 'scientific convention'. After reading, or better, writing a few pages from which the excess has been cut, one soon develops a taste for this type of surgery. The outcome of excision is shorter, clearer text with a sense of coming to the point.

> *(IT) HAS BEEN SHOWN (THAT)...*
>
> *(IT) HAS BEEN FOUND (THAT)...*
>
> *(IT) WAS NOTED (THAT)...*
>
> *(IT) WAS SHOWN TO BE, etc.*

These constructions can usually be omitted or replaced by a simple verb.

> It has been shown that plasma cholinesterase is decreased in pregnancy...
>
> It has been shown that [some drugs] cause a fall in plasma potassium...

Make the unqualified statements: *plasma cholinesterase is decreased in pregnancy; [some drugs] cause a fall in plasma potassium.* Many writers use *it has been shown that* to imply doubt but if there is doubt about the universality of an observation it is better to be explicit. The constructions can be avoided completely by writing *Smith's group showed that*, which avoids the implication that the observation is universal.

They have been shown to be remarkably reliable when used in this way.

They *are* reliable when used in this way. If you think or know they aren't reliable, then say so.

One patient was noted to have a number of polyps. . .

One patient *had* a number of polyps.

At the time of intubation it was noted that. . .

It was noted that is unnecessary unless the report is written by someone who was not there at the time and who has obtained the information from the patient's notes.

. . .the tracheal wall was found to be harder than normal. . .

The tracheal wall *was* harder than normal.

Increased longevity, as well as symptomatic relief, is reported to follow surgical correction. . .

Longevity *follows* surgical correction, but the whole construction is clumsy (and see FOLLOWING). *Surgical correction prolongs life and relieves symptoms* conveys the intended sense.

IN ORDER TO

. . .a flow of 18 L/min is required in order to deliver a tidal volume of. . .

It is sometimes better to write *in order to* (do something), but often the addition of *in order* is just padding.

A sentence that begins *in order to* may be better turned around: *In order to prevent headache, the patients were instructed to remain supine* may be bettter as *The patients were instructed to remain supine to prevent headache.* This often depends on which part of the sentence needs the stress.

WITH RESPECT TO...

WITH REGARD TO...

IN REGARD (TO)...

AS REGARDS...

IN RELATION TO...

IN RESPECT OF...

This type of construction is much overused (see also Expanded to a phrase, p. 126). Sometimes it can be replaced by a preposition; sometimes there is a better choice of verb (see CONCERN, REGARD); sometimes it is superfluous. It is a good indicator of poor writing.

Versions of the phrase tend to occur in opening paragraphs of Results sections where the writers describe the patients enlisted to the study.

> The groups were broadly comparable with respect to age and weight.

The groups were of comparable ages and weights is less pompous. SIMILAR would be better than COMPARABLE.

> The two groups of patients did not differ significantly with respect to age, sex and weight.

It is awkward to write of two groups having similar sexes. Try: *Ages, weights and sex ratios were similar for the two groups.* Often, the text repeats the contents of a table:

> Table I shows that the two groups of patients were broadly comparable with respect to age, gender, weight and duration of bypass.

> Details of the patients studied are shown in Table I. There was no difference between the groups with respect to age, body weight, body type, duration of preoperative starvation and duration of surgery.

> There were no statistical differences between the groups with respect to age, sex and weight (Table I).

If there is a table, the easiest way to avoid the construction is to write something like: *There were no significant clinical differences between the two groups before surgery (Table I).*

This will make the paper shorter and easier to read (as will deleting other repetition between tables and text – a particularly common fault and one that annoys astute reviewers and editors, not least because 'Instructions to Authors' are often specific in excluding this habit).

Note the capital letter in references to a particular figure or table: *Figure 3, Table IV.*

> We have been unable to determine accurately the site of the stenosis in relation to the anastomosis in all cases from the [survey details].

Here *in relation to* is used correctly to indicate physical proximity, but the sentence reads awkwardly and is ambiguous. The writers meant that they were able to determine the site in most cases, but the sentence could be read to mean that they were unable to determine the site in any of the cases. Try: *From the [survey details], we could not always be certain how near the stenosis was to the anastomosis.*

It would not be correct to write *We have been unable to determine the correct relation of the stenosis to the anastomosis* because this does not define whether the relation is anatomical or aetiological.

Finding one of these constructions is often an indication that the sentence is the wrong way round. Inverting the sentence then allows deletion of the superfluous phrase and makes expression of the ideas more direct:

> The fact that anaesthetists are no different from other doctors in relation to accurate record keeping need not be an occasion for surprise. . .

Anaesthetists keep records no more accurately than do other doctors, which is no surprise. . .

> There remains a dearth of comparisons with traditional methods in respect of effectiveness, safety and feasibility.

There have been few studies in which its effectiveness, safety and feasibility have been compared with traditional methods.

> . . .there is geographical variation in the natural history of stomach cancer as regards metastatic spread to the liver. . .

The geographical variation is not of metastasis but of the incidence of metastasis, so . . .*the incidence of metastatic spread of stomach cancer to the liver shows geographical variation. . ..*

The example can be improved further: . . . *is different in different countries (or counties, or continents)* is neater and gives more information than *shows geographical variation.*

IN THE CASE OF, IS THE CASE, see CASE and p. 96

IN TERMS OF

This expression is best used for a mathematical description of one variable in terms of another variable or variables. It can be a useful device but should not be overused. The tendency is to write *in terms of* to introduce each comparison: *in terms of operating time. . ., in terms of ease of closure. . ., in terms of infection rate. . . .*

> In terms of stoma management, there seems little difference between a colostomy and an ileostomy as assessed in this trial.

This trial showed that colostomies and ileostomies were equally easy to manage conveys the sense.

> In terms of depression, it has been found that men take longer to recover from the loss of a partner than women.

'It has been found that' is superfluous (see above): *Men are depressed for longer than women after loss of their partners.*

> This is an advantage in terms of reduced operative time, hospital stay and patient morbidity.

The advantage can be described *in terms of operative time*, but not in terms of *reduced* operative time – that *is* the advantage. At the least, *in terms of* should be replaced by *because of;* an improvement, but the sentence still reads awkwardly because *reduced* applies also (understood) to *hospital stay* and *patient morbidity.*

There is a better choice of words: *This is an advantage because operating time is reduced, stay in hospital is shorter, and there is less morbidity. Operating* time is better than *operative* time. The *stay* was not by the hospital but by the patients in hospital (see Nouns as adjectives, p. 162): *patient* morbidity is unnecessary.

Some would argue that *morbidity* is used as a catch-all here. We don't think the simple substitution of *illness* or *disease* would work, but something more explicit like *less conducive to postoperative illness* might be preferable.

> The study has highlighted that there is no difference in terms of wound healing between either method. . .

. . .*wounds heal equally well with both methods.* . . .. The writers have made the not uncommon error of writing of a 'difference . . . between either method'. Differences exist *between one and another* but not *between either one or another* (see pp. 103 and 124).

HIGHLIGHTING is something you do with a pen containing fluorescent ink: depending on the context *shown* or *confirmed* is better (see p. 111).

(by) the USE OF

(by) the PRESENCE OF

(by) the FINDING OF

> The use of regional analgesia may [cause] greater heat loss. . .

> . . .by the presence of the fixed leak. . .

> Most important must be the presence of close liaison between surgeon and physician.

Something cannot have any effect if it is not used or is absent; these phrases are padding (see also expansions of *by*, p. 127) and are better omitted altogether. One meaning of *liaison* is (*COD*) an illicit sexual relationship. Unless that is what is meant, *Surgeon and physician must work closely together* is better.

> It may be asked if one would be prepared to operate on the mother's history alone in the absence of any positive signs of a hernia.

In the absence of, which in plain English is *if there are no,* is not the only fault here. The awkward *It may be asked if.* . . is better as a direct question *Should you.* . .?. The order of the ideas suggests it is the mother's history that is due for operation. Try: *Should you operate if a mother describes a hernia, but you can find no signs of one?*

Other words can be misused similarly. *We have confirmed the finding of.* . . is better as *We have confirmed that.* . .; *This method has the capability of.* . . and *They have the capacity to.* . . are better as *This method can.* . . and *They can.* . . (see p. 53).

Other examples of repetition

An item was advertised in a pamphlet on road safety as 'red in colour'. This is equivalent to writing that patients were *tall in height* or *heavy in weight* and when put plainly like this is plainly nonsense. However:

> The duration of the operating session was calculated to be the time between. . .

A duration can be taken, or calculated, *as* the time between two events, but it cannot be calculated *to be* that time. The duration actually *was* that time, which makes the phrase *calculated to be* superfluous.

> For each relaxant the ascending EC_{50} was close in value to the descending EC_{50} and there was no significant difference between them.

When commenting on this, it is difficult not to be sarcastic. Perhaps the EC_{50} (a comparative measure of the drug dose) was close in emotional terms? The comment about significance compounds the error by repetition. Re-arrangement gives: *For each relaxant there were no significant differences between the ascending and descending EC_{50},* or better *There were no significant differences between the ascending and descending EC_{50} values for any of the relaxants.*

8
Trouble with short words

Many short words can act as different parts of speech: prepositions, conjunctions, adverbs or pronouns (see p. 29). Instead of being grouped grammatically, the words are grouped here under more general headings to make it easier to find and correct mistakes.

Following a verb

Certain verbs are followed by particular prepositions. Some verbs alter their meanings with the preposition; *compare* is the verb most misused in this way. It can be helpful when trying to decide which preposition is correct to consider the nouns formed from the verbs (and vice versa). For instance, which is correct of *different from*, *different to* and *different than*? Most people using *to differ* say *it differs from*; thus *different* is usually followed by *from* not *to*. (*Different than* is American usage.)

COMPARE *to or with?*

Compare to means *liken to*. The example usually quoted is from Shakespeare's sonnet: 'Shall I compare thee to a summer's day?' A comparison between one thing and another (or a number of others) is always one *with* another. *Compare with* also allows the consideration of both similarities and differences.

> . . .lower after epidural compared to intraperitoneal. . .

> This is not a great drawback when compared to the use of musculocutaneous flaps. . .

Both should be *compared with* (but see use of *than* below).

Drawback is not a good choice of word, particularly when discussing flaps. There is the joke:

> 'What is the biggest drawback in the jungle?'
> 'An elephant's foreskin.'

Disadvantage is the required word.

> Transfused patients had a poorer prognosis compared to non-transfused patients. . .

Again this should be *compared with* but it is neater to replace *compared to* with *than*.

Patients are not transfused; blood is transfused into them. No one would write *infused patients* to mean patients given an infusion of fluid. This is part of the tendency to turn nouns into verbs: patients are bronchoscoped, endoscoped, coronary artery bypass grafted. We have seen the noun *increment* converted to a verb *to increment* used in the sense *giving incremental doses*. This is a habit to avoid because it is slovenly and almost always a sign of a lazy writer. Worse, the habit can cause ambiguity. Although no one is likely to misunderstand *The patient was coronary artery bypass grafted*, the similar *We digitalized the patient* could 'imply a rectal examination, or a binary transformation of the patient'.[35]

There is no need to repeat the phrase *blood transfusion* once it is established what exactly was transfused (e.g. whole blood, platelets, white cells). The above example is better as: *Patients who received a transfusion had a worse prognosis*; or *Patients to whom blood had been given had a worse prognosis*; but best is *Transfusion worsened prognosis*.

> There is a. . .difference between the incidence of clinical as compared to radiological leak rates. . .

This is a more complex error. There can be a difference *between* one item *and another* item; it is incorrect to write of a difference *between one* item *compared with another* item – unless the items are themselves differences between other pairs of entities (see pp. 103 and 121). The example should read . . .*difference between the incidence of leak rates detected clinically and radiologically* to be correct. Even when 'compared with' (or to) is used correctly there is no need to precede the phrase with 'as', a common superfluity in this type of construction.

The usual error is compared *to* written in error for compared *with*, but not always.

> The function of the cobalt in B_{12} can be compared with that of the iron in haemoglobin. . .

The writer was pointing out a similarity, and *compared to* is required. FUNCTION is correct here (see p. 81). If *function* is omitted, readers will not know if the writer is referring to some other property, such as position or state of ionization.

CONNECT to or with?

> Each model consists of a linear resistance connected in series with a compliance.

Connect is always followed by *to* not *with*. This example can be simplified further: if the model is a resistance and a compliance, then these components must be connected. *Each model consists of* (or COMPRISES) *a linear resistance in series with a compliance.*

DEFINE by or as?

> Toxic dilatation was defined by the radiographic demonstration of gas. . .

Here the writers are saying that radiographic demonstration is the equivalent of toxic dilatation, that the one is the same as the other: toxic dilatation was defined *as*. . .. This equivalence is defined *by* the writers. (See DILATION/DILATATION.)

Demonstration is not a good choice (see p. 57); *defined*, depending on the context, might be better replaced by *diagnosed*. An improved version of the example is *Toxic dilatation was diagnosed from the radiographic appearance of gas*. . .. But, in another context, *The extent of toxic dilatation was defined by*. . . would have conveyed an accurate meaning, with *defined* meaning *marked out, delineated*.

REPLACE with or by?

SUBSTITUTE with, by or for?

Replace means *take the place of*. Either *with* or *by* can be correct, so both *We replaced plaster of Paris with acrylic* and *We replaced plaster of Paris by acrylic* are acceptable.

Substitute means *put in the place of,* and the correct preposition is *for*: *We substituted acrylic for plaster of Paris.*

SEDATE with or by?

TREAT with or by?

Either word can be used. A journal may have an editorial preference, so you may find your choice changed by the sub-editor. For consistency, use *with* if the treatment is an object, a drug for example:

> . . .adequately sedated with morphine. . .

and *by* if it is an action:

> . . .treated by a course of physiotherapy. . .

> . . .treated by renewal of the pacing wire. . .

Expanded to a phrase

Medical writers frequently expand prepositions and conjunctions into phrases. Many expansions are common enough for it to be worthwhile searching for them by word processor.

IN THE CASE OF

There is never need to use this construction. Its use is a sign of laziness: the writer either has not looked for a better word or has constructed the sentence poorly. This example is from a journal's 'Guide to contributors'.

> In the case of books, the references should be as follows:. . .

In the case of can be replaced by *for*, though *References to books should be as follows:* is better.

> Except in the case of the oldest and youngest, all the children. . .

Again *for* is the replaced preposition. *Except for the oldest. . .* is good; better is to turn the sentence around: *All the children, except the oldest. . ..*

WITH RESPECT TO

> This is considerably less than the previous recommendations with respect to the Lack breathing system.

Simply *for.* (See also p. 129.)

BY MEANS OF. . .

BY VIRTUE OF. . .

. . .is by means of a T-piece system. . .

. . .by means of various pretreatments.

. . .kept in contact by virtue of the considerable forces. . .

These are expansions of *by.* The preposition alone is sufficient.

IN CONJUNCTION WITH

. . .this arrangement cannot be used in conjunction with a flow generator. . .

With implies a conjunction, a joining, of two objects; *in conjunction* is unnecessary.

AS TO

This common construction is sometimes justified. It is often superfluous – particularly before when, who, what, how and whether (Phythian, *A Concise Dictionary of Correct English*, pp. 15–6). It is also used instead of single prepositions.

. . .accurate information as to our future needs and our present inefficiencies.

The correct preposition here is *about.*

. . .a relatively good indicator as to whether the procedure is likely to be useful.

Replacing *as to* by *of* is an improvement but the sentence is clumsy. Try: . . . *a relatively good indicator of the usefulness of the procedure.*

. . .and obviously raises the question as to whether it should be the primary method. . .

as to could be replaced by *of.* Better is . . .*and obviously suggests that it might not be the best primary method.*

Variations of because

Because: defined by the *COD* as by reason of, on account of, for the reason that.

AS, SINCE, FOR
DUE TO, OWING TO
BY REASON OF (the fact that)
IN VIEW OF (the fact that)
The reason is because (of) the fact that

All of these are used to mean *because*: to introduce a subordinate idea, a rider, to the main clause. A single word is almost always preferable to a longer construction.

We have the impression that *because* is gradually disappearing from medical writing. Could this be because it incorporates the terrible word *cause*? Caution in attributing causality may be praiseworthy in any science but using *because* does not imply anything but a most general type of this attribution. And anyway all the alternatives do the same, but less accurately or more euphemistically.

As and *since* may introduce ambiguity by implying a temporal relation. (Some editors reserve *since* as a temporal descriptor, but many writers don't appreciate this nicety.)

As I gave the injection, the patient collapsed can mean either *Because I gave. . .* or *While I was giving. . ..* The required meaning is made clear by using *because*, or by inverting the sentence to put the main clause first: *The patient collapsed as I gave the injection* means that the patient collapsed while I was injecting.

Since I had given the injection, the patient had collapsed is similarly ambiguous: the collapse may have been my fault, or I may simply be describing the order of events. *Because* makes it clear that it was my fault; inverting the sentence makes it clear that, for whatever reason, the collapse occurred after the injection.

It is accepted usage to write *as* and *since* to mean *because*, but one should be aware of these possible ambiguities. Using *because* usually prevents confusion.

Because can be ambiguous with negatives. Note the meanings of the next two examples, and the difference the comma makes.

> *The incision did not dehisce because nylon sutures were used* [it dehisced because of something else].

> *The incision did not dehisce, because nylon sutures were used* [and they prevent dehiscence].

Writing the subordinate clause first (*Because nylon sutures were used,*) expresses the second of these meanings, and stresses the type of suture rather than the lack of dehiscence.

For is used mainly by literary writers as a way of emphasizing the subordinate clause. Medical writers do not tend to use *for* to mean *because.*

With the exception of *owing to* and sometimes of *due to* (see below), all the other constructions are better replaced by *because* or *because of.* Appending *the fact that* or even wordier constructions – *the reason is because of the fact that* – is unnecessary: *because* suffices.

SINCE

> Since the incidence of awareness is low, a large number of patients would be required. . .

Since is acceptable here. The present tense in the opening, subordinate, clause indicates that *since* means *because* and not *from the time that.* The main idea is of the need for a large number of patients, and the opening clause is a rider to this: *since* meaning *because* is accepted usage. *Because* is better though.

> It is a sensible change since no longer can individuals acquire the wide and deep experience to cover the whole field. . .

Since has both its senses and is acceptable. . . .*because one person can no longer be expected to cover the whole field* is better though.

> General anaesthetic techniques were rejected since they can cause cardiovascular upset.

Since is incorrect. General anaesthesia has always been liable to depress the cardiovascular system: use *as* or *because.* A better overall construction is *General anaesthesia was unsuitable because. . ..*

> . . .these should not be used for the subclavian route since distortion of the catheter can. . .

Again, *as* or *because.*

DUE TO/OWING TO

Due is an adjective, as in *The rent is due.* It cannot be used as an adverb. There is a correct use of *due to* (see below) but this construction is used, rightly and wrongly, to such excess in medical writing that to search and replace it might be regarded as a duty. The first is a typical example:

> This first study was abandoned due to poor patient compliance.

This is incorrect because *due* is then adverbial, qualifying *abandoned* (a past participle of a verb, acting as an adjective). Writing *The abandonment of the study was due to. . .* is grammatically correct because *due* is adjectival, qualifying *abandonment* (a noun), but it is clumsy. Because of this point of grammar, it is best to avoid using *due to* to mean *because of.*

Owing *to* can be substituted for *due to* in the above example, and *owing to poor compliance by the patients* avoids the use of *patient* as an adjective (see Nouns as adjectives, p. 162).

> These improved results from Japan may be due in part to the large screening programmes. . .

Due describes the results, and is correct; although one could just as easily write *partly because of. . . .*

> The free gift in this packet is unsuitable for children under 3 years, due to small parts.

Not written by a doctor this time; the packet was a packet of breakfast cereal and it was the free gift, not the children, that had the small parts. Replacing *due to* with *because of* or *owing to* fails to remove the ambiguity; the sentence needs rewriting: *Because it contains small parts, the free gift in this packet is unsuitable for children under 3 years.* Even when rewritten, this warning – intended presumably to stop children inhaling a chunk of plastic – is fairly insipid. Why not: *Danger of choking! Free gift not for children under 3!* This is no more grammatical than the original, but warnings are supposed to be effective, not grammatically correct.

As an aside, this observation about ineffectual instructions and warnings is a general one, certainly prevalent in the instruction leaflets that come with drugs and medical equipment. Here is the second paragraph of warnings from a leaflet insert for equipment used only in minimally invasive procedures:

> Minimally invasive instruments may vary in diameter from manufacturer
> to manufacturer. When minimally invasive instruments and accessories
> from different manufacturers are employed together in a procedure,
> verify compatibility prior to initiation of the procedure.

Bearing in mind that the whole leaflet was about minimally invasive procedures, and that the first paragraph contained the phrase 'minimally
invasive' three times, why was the phrase necessary even once? Is this
another medicolegal influence on the language (see p. 20)? This instruction
is saying, 'Check things fit together before you start!' Note EMPLOYED,
INITIATION, the repetition of *procedure*, and *verify* preferred to *check*.

> None of the differences were [sic] statistically significant due to
> marked variation. . .

> . . ., although due to small numbers the figures did not reach
> statistical significance.

Due to is grammatically incorrect: in the first example it is qualifying the
adjective *significant*, in the second the verb *reach*. Replace by *because of*, or
owing to.

There is a more serious error implicit in these examples. It is common
to find writers stating that their results did not reach significance because
of small numbers, marked variation or some similar explanation, but it
shows a misunderstanding of inferential statistics. Perhaps more patients,
or less variation, would have brought out a difference; but it may also be
that there is no difference. Writers must not use incomplete results to
support their favoured notions (see pp. 5 and 18). This is not the place
for discussion of type II (beta) error; readers should consult books on
statistics for further explanation.

Another misuse of language in the presentation of statistics is writing
the pulse rate remained constant to mean *the pulse rate did not change
significantly*: they are not synonymous. Something can be constant only if
it does not change at all, for example the pulse rate in a patient with a
cardiac pacemaker set to deliver a fixed rate.

ON ACCOUNT OF

BY REASON OF

These phrases are the dictionary definition of *because* and should be
replaced by the single word.

All patients underwent induction of labour on account of postmaturity.

. . .not suitable on account of pelvic floor dysfunction.

Replace with *because of. Pelvic floor dysfunction* is better as *dysfunction of the pelvic floor.*

IN VIEW OF

. . .in view of the discrepancy between. . .

This is a metaphorical use of *view. In view of* is a flowery way of writing *because of,* though it is reasonable if the sense is *bearing in mind that. Flowery* is itself a metaphor for complicated (see Metaphor, p. 156).

THAT, WHICH, WHEN, WHERE, WHEREBY

These words relate one thing or idea with another, or refer back to a place, time or thing that has already been mentioned. They are difficult words grammatically (depending on the construction they can be adverbs, conjunctions or pronouns), but choice of the best word does not depend on knowing the precise part of speech.

THAT/WHICH

Consider these two sentences.

1 The studies that they reported were ethical.
2 The studies, which they reported, were ethical.

Sentence 1 states that the reported studies were ethical but implies there are other unreported studies that were not. *That they reported* is a *defining clause,* known grammatically as a restrictive clause, and deleting it alters the meaning of the sentence in an important way. Sentence 2 is a simple statement that the studies were ethical. *Which they reported* is a *describing clause,* grammatically it is non-restrictive, and it is not essential to the meaning.

Another pair of examples is:

1 Do not give steroids that are diabetogenic.
2 Do not give steroids, which are diabetogenic.

Sentence 1 allows you to give steroids, provided they are the particular steroids that do not cause diabetes; sentence 2 forbids all steroids because steroids cause diabetes.

> The two studies were open to two types of bias. Both relied on a clinical diagnosis which can be unreliable.

The intended meaning was that *both studies were unreliable* because they relied on the diagnosis, not that the clinical diagnosis itself can be unreliable: a comma is needed before *which*. Another ambiguity is that *both* could mean *both* studies or *both* types of bias (see p. 179); writing *Both studies* (the intended meaning) avoids this ambiguity.

In general, defining clauses should start with *that* and describing clauses with *which*. There is not strict agreement on this, despite what some grammarians maintain, but *that* must not introduce a describing clause, and describing clauses must always be marked off from the main clause, usually by commas but sometimes by parentheses.

To put it another way, if your sentence and its meaning survive intact on removing the which/that clause, then the clause should have begun with *which* and it should have been punctuated parenthetically. A few publishers and rather more sub-editors make a rigorous distinction between the use of *which* and *that* in all rather than in just essential circumstances. This is a good thing because of removing all ambiguity, but it is problematical because even the part of the argument that constitutes the rule is poorly understood and widely disobeyed, which provides the aggrieved writer with numerous quotations from respectable sources in support of the chosen usage. This is all made more difficult by the freely interchangeable way *which* and *that* are used in speech. To return to a noble example (see p. 25):

> This structure has novel features which are of considerable biological interest.

Watson and Crick[21] wrote *which* where *that* technically might have been preferable though not obligatory (but did the structure have other novel but uninteresting features?). Watson is American, and Americans tend to prefer *which* (the older form in this instance). A comma after *features* would have made *that* incorrect and reinforced *which*. As Watson and Crick wrote it, the *which* clause is not parenthetically embedded and, if spoken, the sentence might have been broken by a 'breath', a slight pause, after *features.* We see no reason why *which* in this context should not carry implicit punctuation like *and, but* and other conjunctions.

> **Cavernous sinus thrombosis is a rare complication of orbital cellulitis, which has a high morbidity.**

It is cavernous sinus thrombosis that has the high morbidity; whether *which* or *that* is preferred, there should not be a comma.

Confusion, overuse and misuse of *that* and *which* often occur because writers are concerned about repeating the original noun, choosing instead to write a longer sentence joined by *that* or *which.* Meaning may be clearer with repetition. Watson and Crick repeated *structure* to good effect (see p. 25). The belief that repeating words is always poor style is misplaced. So-called 'elegant variation' is often anything but.

Long sentences that include numerous clauses introduced by *that* and *which* read awkwardly and readers may be uncertain of the connections between the pronouns and nouns (see p. 170).

> **The higher dose produced complications, of which the most important was radiation pneumonitis, which is frequently lethal.**

The problem with writing about *complications, of which. . ., which. . .* is that readers may not know what is being referred to. Although re-reading may enable readers to understand, sentences should be clear and unambiguous on first reading. Bryson believes that 'No reader should ever be required to retrace his steps, however short the journey.' Try: *The higher dose had complications including radiation pneumonitis, which is the most important as it is frequently lethal.*

Sometimes *that* can be dropped altogether (an example of ellipsis, see p. 162): *The argument [that] we make. . ..* But, taking an example from the sentence before the last quotation, replacing *Long sentences that include numerous clauses. . .* with *Long sentences including numerous clauses. . .* is neither elegant nor quite correct, though many give way to the temptation.

WHEN, WHERE/AT or IN WHICH

> **. . .techniques where increasing concentrations are given. . .**

Where has connotations of place; *when* has connotations of time. Use *at which* or *in which* (correct for the example) if there are no connotations of either.

WHEREBY/THEREBY

Whereby means *as result of which* or *by which means* and so is incorrect in:

> [It should have] the means whereby the inspired gases may be warmed and humidified. . .

Whereby is overused; *by which* or *in which* is usually better. In the example, it is a pointer to generally poor style. Try: *[It should have] a way of warming and humidifying the inspired gases.*

Thereby means *as result of that* or *by that means*. It may be better replaced with the simpler *this* or *that*.

Words of comment: THEREFORE, HOWEVER and others

Use sparingly. Medical writers tend to start alternate sentences with one of these words – particularly in the Discussion sections of papers – and *however* is especially common because it usually precedes an explanation of why the writers' conclusions are at variance with previous work.

Therefore and *thus* can often be deleted; take readers along with you by logical development of ideas. *However* can often be replaced by combining two sentences by *but* or *although*. Some authorities hold that a sentence must never start with *however* while others disagree. Whichever is held as correct, *however* is overused in medical writing.

However beginning a sentence, with the meaning, 'That having been said', must be followed by a comma. *However we did it. . .*, in which *however* means '*In whatever way*' and is not followed by a comma, means something different from *However, we did it. . ..*

> However these amounts of tilt are probably infrequently used, even if intended.

> However acceptance of death is denied or delayed, the human body is inexorably destined to decay. . ..

The first example is incorrect and needs a comma after *However*; the second is correct and must not have a comma.

However refutes – *However, Brown used small groups of patients and did not measure the cardiac output* – indeed reinforces – *Brown's study was flawed, indeed the samples were small and he did not measure cardiac output.*

Few would use *indeed* in speech; it is an affected word that should be used sparingly in writing.

These words, others are *moreover, nevertheless* and *nonetheless*, (which some insist is three words *none the less*) are all words that emphasize, and too much emphasis loses effect.

Words of reference: FORMER AND LATTER, RESPECTIVELY, SUCH

FORMER and LATTER

Former and *latter* are correct only for a list of two items; for a list of more than two, *first* and *last* are correct. *Former* and *latter* often indicate clumsy writing and can be omitted, or avoided by rephrasing. Particularly careful editors ban *former* and *latter* constructions because they confuse and make the reader back-track.

> Initial treatment can be with saline, Hartmann's solution, or plasma substitutes. If the latter are used. . .

It is better here to repeat *plasma substitutes*. Starting the second sentence instead with *If these are used* does not define whether *these* are *plasma substitutes* alone or *saline, Hartmann's solution and plasma substitutes.*

> However, when comparisons are made between controlled clinical trials and the reports of adverse reactions in the literature, a much greater frequency of anaphylactoid reactions is encountered in the former.

This is a typically confused piece of medical prose. *Former* is grammatically correct, referring to the first of *controlled clinical trials* and *reports of adverse reactions*. But surely 'the literature' (a misnomer if ever there was one, see p. 7) *includes* controlled clinical trials? Presumably, by writing of *reports of adverse reactions* the writers are alluding to case reports. What the writers should have written is *More anaphylactoid reactions are reported during controlled clinical trials than is suggested by reading case reports,* which actually seems unlikely. What failure of education makes intelligent people write in this contorted way?

> The tracheal wall was thin, with atrophied muscular and elastic tissue. This may lead to tracheobronchial collapse with signs of chronic infection. The latter can result in respiratory insufficiency and cor pulmonale.

What is *latter* referring to? Again, this example needs rewriting. The chain of events from the thin tracheal wall to cor pulmonale is not made clear.

It is clearer as *The tracheal wall, with atrophied muscle and elastic tissue, was thin. This may lead to tracheobronchial collapse, chronic infection and eventually to respiratory insufficiency and cor pulmonale.*

RESPECTIVELY

This is a useful word with which to identify the correct connections between items in lists, but it can usually be omitted.

Respectively is correct in *The doses of penicillin, cloxacillin, and flucloxacillin are 600 mg, 500 mg, and 250 mg, respectively,* but the sentence is better as *The doses are 600 mg penicillin, 500 mg cloxacillin, and 250 mg flucloxacillin.*

Respectively must be preceded by a comma.

> Some responses did not recover completely, 90% and 100% recovery were not reached by one and six cases respectively.

One case did not recover to 90% and six cases did not recover to 100% is better. Under most circumstances, *recover to 100%* is better as *recover completely.*

> The mean ages of groups A and B were 35.6 and 37.2 years respectively.

> Injury mortality fell for children in every social class, although the decline for children in social classes I and II (32% and 37% respectively) was greater than for children in social classes IV and V (21% and 2% respectively).

Respectively is only necessary if there could be ambiguity. There is unlikely to be confusion with lists of two, and respectively can be omitted in both examples. *Fewer children died of their injuries* is better than 'injury mortality fell for children'.

SUCH

Such means *this and similar* or *these and similar. Such* should not be used instead of *this* or *these.*

> Better management has led to an improved survival of those with severe disease, and it is usually such patients who develop. . .

Such patients are simply those with severe disease, the writers did not intend those with severe disease *and other similar patients. Such* should be *these*.

> Day-case units are becoming more common. One group of patients who would certainly benefit from such a facility would be those who undergo diagnostic endoscopy.

From such a facility can be omitted.

> As with all new products and procedures there are points of detail that are important if full advantage is to be derived from such an innovation.

Such an should be *this*, but this sentence is repetitive because an innovation is something newly introduced. Either *As with all new products and procedures. . .* or *. . .from this innovation.*

Such in the construction *such as* is a more elegant way of writing *e.g.*:

> . . .is most effective in a tumour with a relatively long natural history, such as carcinoma of the prostate. . .

(*Relatively* could be omitted with no loss of meaning.)

The use of *e.g.* and *i.e.* in medical writing is so excessive that it is worth pointing out that there are non-medical publishers who insist upon these being written as *for example* and *that is* in every instance. (This would certainly prevent writers putting *i.e.* when they actually mean *e.g.*, a not uncommon error.) Some publishers even have *et cetera* spelled out. We assume from this behaviour that their writers are also expected to use the numerous and preferable alternatives. It would not be too arduous for medical writers to do the same (see Avoiding abbreviations, p. 188).

9
Use of the passive voice

Using the active, we write, 'He made the incision. . .' using the passive, 'The incision was made. . .'. An established but not absolute convention (see p. 150) was for all scientific writing to be in the passive voice.

> Nor need we be deceived by the impersonal passive voice in which such messages [scientific communication] are conventionally cast. . . The fundamental principle of scientific observation is that all human beings are interchangeable as observers.[36]

Unfortunately, this allegedly fundamental principle (which is increasingly open to question) also makes scientific writing ugly and unwieldy. It is to some extent a matter of fashion, but fashion is now turning against the passive.

When the passive voice is used, the writers take a back seat, as if they had watched the study from a distance: *It was decided to*; *three measurements were taken*. The passive forces constructions such as *It was necessary to* and *This necessitated* instead of *We had to*. Medical writers may be reluctant to use the active voice because of a fear that the first person sounds somehow immodest. Used sensibly it does not, but it does lend a paper a directness that gives readers the sense that the writers actually did the work, or hold the opinions, that they describe.

> We discussed the therapeutic potential of fish oil in an editorial last year.

This, the first sentence from an unsigned editorial in the *Lancet*, is more effective than the passive equivalent *The therapeutic potential of fish oil was discussed in an editorial in this journal last year.*

> If thought is given to the [many underlying] factors, unnecessary surgery can be avoided.

There is no need for surgery.

The passive, sometimes called *the third person*, can be a useful device if a paper has several writers, each of whom did a particular part of the study, but it is still best to avoid long series of sentences in which this was noted and that was measured. Apart from anything else, it can make the work sound dull and uninteresting.

Many journals insist that abstracts and summaries should not contain first-person statements but this does not mean that the passive need be used throughout these sections of a paper.

There are two, contrasting, occasions when the passive may be better. The doer of an action may be unimportant: *The president of the Royal College was honoured yesterday when. . .* stresses the person honoured rather than the person or body of people who did the honouring. Or writers may wish to stress the doers: *The criteria for brain death are checked by two consultants. . ..* This use of the passive plus what is termed a *by-phrase* is also useful when the doer is complicated: *This suggestion was made by the Royal College of Surgeons, the General Medical Council, the Medical Defence Union, The Royal College of Nursing, and Unison* – though the mind boggles at what such a suggestion could be.

Some examples

. . .considerable difficulty was experienced in passing a tube. . .

This was written by the doctor who had the difficulty, and it is better as *I had difficulty passing the tube. . ..*

Was noted is common in passive constructions:

Mobility of the patella was noted in some patients. . .

The shape of the gland was noted and divided into crescentic, semicircular and round.

NOTED in the first example is misused for *noticed*, but it is better to avoid the passive by *Some patients had mobile patellae. . ..*

The second example is imprecise – the shape was *defined* not *divided*; ungrammatical (the shape was crescentic, semicircular *or* round); and repetitive (noting *was* defining). Try: *We defined the shape of the gland as crescentic, semicircular or round.*

Examination of the liver revealed it to be free from obvious metastases.

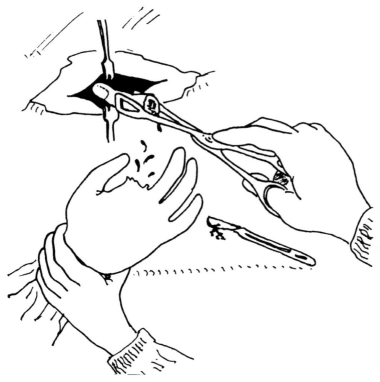

The index finger of the surgeon is then inserted into the atrium.

This means *There were no obvious metastases in the liver.*

> The index finger of the surgeon is then inserted into the atrium. The
> valve is palpated.

The surgeon then puts his finger into the atrium and palpates the valve. You
might wonder who, if not the surgeon, inserts the surgeon's finger into the
atrium. Perhaps the writer wished to avoid the sex bias (see p. 65) of *his* or
the odd-sounding *his or her*, avoiding sex bias by using the indefinite
article (see p. 171) (*puts a finger*) could suggest the digit was acquired
randomly, but surely only to those with a macabre sense of humour.

The verb 'TO PERFORM'

Adherence to the passive voice encourages writers to put *An examination
of the colon was performed* instead of *We examined the colon. The colon is*

examined is good if the passive is preferred. *Perform* is better applied to music and theatre.

Not all the examples below are strictly of the passive, but it is a convenient heading under which to discuss the usage of PERFORM (see also p. 81). Six of these examples are from the same paper – four from the same paragraph.

> Histological examination of the resected colon was performed in every case.

Try *We always examined the resected colon histologically* or, to retain the passive voice, *The resected colon was always examined histologically.*

> Wholegut transit time marker studies were performed in the last 13 patients in the series, and all showed prolonged transit times.

Were performed can be omitted, and the sentence shortened by deleting the repetitions. The inelegant phrase *Wholegut transit time marker studies* is an example of Nouns as adjectives (see p. 162). *Whole gut* should anyway be two words. With these revisions the sentence reads *The times of transit through the whole gut, studied with markers in the last 13 patients, were prolonged.*

> One or other biopsy was performed in *x* of the patients preoperatively, all confirming the presence of ganglia. . .

Omit *was performed* and make more direct: *One or other biopsy, taken preoperatively from x patients, revealed ganglia. Revealed* is better than the shorter *showed* (see p. 88) because the ganglia will not be visible directly but will be brought out by histological stains.

> Motility and pressure studies, performed in *x* patients preoperatively, showed. . .

Preoperative studies of motility and pressure in x *patients showed. . ..*

> In those patients in whom apparently total colectomy was performed. . .

In those patients in whom the colectomy was apparently total. . . Complete would be a better word than *total* except that the operation is described as a *total colectomy.*

> . . . a marker study performed at another hospital showed a normal transit time. However, this latter study was performed after purgation. . .

Omit and combine the sentences: . . .*a marker study, at another hospital, showed a normal time, although this was after purgation* (see LATTER).

> It has been suggested that venography should be performed in all cases (Smith, 1985).

This example has two passive constructions: *it has been suggested that* and *should be performed*. They can be avoided by putting the writer first: *Smith (1985) suggested venography in all cases*. If Smith suggested that venography was essential, then *essential* is the correct word: *Smith (1985) suggested venography was essential*. This is more emphatic than *in all cases*.

> Gynaecological patients can now expect to have their operations performed in the day unit within two weeks.

Patients are not gynaecological. Patients have gynaecological diseases and they are admitted to hospital for gynaecological operations. A particular hate of one of us is 'head-injured patients': these are *patients with head injuries*.

Omit *performed* (and *to have*): *Patients waiting for gynaecological operations can now expect to be admitted to the day unit within two weeks*.

Some points of style raised by this example will be discussed again in the sections on word order. The example is from a paper discussing the advantages of a unit for day-case surgery. The writers should be stressing that the patients will have their operations sooner, but the construction of their sentence stresses that the operations will take place in the day unit.

Conclusion

How should we sum up the use of the passive voice, probably the most ubiquitous marker of conventional scientific medical style? Is the passive voice something intrinsic to good style? We hold that it is only a convention, and often a damaging one. The replacement of passive with active constructions, using personal pronouns where necessary and with effective use of references, makes writing simple and clear.

Two main arguments are put forward by those who criticize the replacing of embellishments like *It has been suggested that. . .* with short, active constructions. The first criticism of what they regard as over-zealous editing is that it makes the text too sparse and arid. This is sometimes true, but bearing in mind the amount of written matter that medical readers have to get through (or think they have to get through), give us sparseness every time.

The second criticism is more important, and more insidious: that what we describe as mostly padding is in fact a way of introducing subtleties of meaning. To take *It has been suggested that*. . . as an example, it is obvious that in speech this could be stressed in a number of ways. One form of accentuation could lead the listener to understand that what is meant is *it has been suggested (but I don't believe a word of it because that lot always cook their results) that*. . ..

The same cannot be managed in writing without using more and explicit words. It is a nonsense to suggest that phrases of this sort, which are otherwise superfluous, have, by their repetition, been encoded with universally understandable nuances of meaning (but see p. 150).

10

Consistency: number and tenses

Number: singular or plural?

Errors in which singular subjects govern plural verbs, or vice versa, are examples of what grammarians refer to as errors of *concord*. Concord – agreement – between subject and verb is the most important type. Mistakes occur most commonly with *either. . .or, neither. . .nor, none*, in lists, and with collective nouns (particularly when the noun is separated from the verb by a long clause). The error that many people seem to know about, but that is the least important, is the one made with the word DATA.

EITHER. . .OR, NEITHER. . .NOR, EACH

In *Either Mr A is a liar or Mrs B is psychotic* the verb is repeated and there is no confusion: the verb is singular. It is also singular if *one or the other* is the subject of the same verb: *Either Mr A or Mrs B is psychotic.*

> Neither thiopental or methohexital are ideal induction agents.

Neither one *nor* (*either* links with *or*; *neither* with *nor*) the other *is* an ideal induction agent. These constructions cannot be applied to more than two choices.

When one of the choices is singular and the other plural, write the plural noun second: *Neither the doctor nor the nurses are responsible. . ..* The plural noun then governs the verb by the *principle of proximity.*

In speech, the plural is more natural when *either. . .or* or *neither. . .nor* is used.

Each implies a consideration of things taken one at a time and is singular: *Each patient was asked. . ..* The mistake is likely with the construction *Each of the patients. . .* when *were* is more natural but *was* is correct. Correcting the error of style (*. . .of the. . .* is unnecessary) makes the mistake less likely and is a good example of how good style can lead naturally to correct grammar.

> Five adult mice were sacrificed and the sternum and all costal cartilage up to the costo-chondral junction were removed in one piece.

There is confusion between the five mice and single specimens of grouped material taken from each mouse. The clearest way of expressing this is *were removed from each in one piece*. (Also see SACRIFICE.)

NONE, ANY, ALL

None means *not one* or *not any* and takes the singular.

> None of the drugs [not one of them] was prescribed.

> None of the drug [not any of it] was prescribed.

All and *any* take the plural if qualifying number and the singular if qualifying amount.

> All of the drugs were prescribed.

> All of the drug was prescribed.

Lists

Lists that include *and* take the plural; lists that include *or* take the singular.

> Its incidence and severity appears to be rising.

> The synchronous development of this apparatus and improved techniques in access to the kidney has led to a revolution. . .

The first should be *appear* (though *seem* is a better word). The second should be *have*. When run through the grammar checker of a well-known word-processing program, neither of these examples provoked correction. We wonder if this anomaly is responsible for what seems to be a rising tide of errors of agreement of this kind.

Synchronous implies an orchestrated development, whereas the development of each had merely taken place over the same period: *The development of this apparatus has coincided with improved methods of access to the kidney, and this has led to a revolution. . ...* The pronoun *this* is now singular, because it refers to *development*, not to *apparatus and access.*

> The age, weight, height and premedication–induction interval were similar for the three groups.

Here the plural verb *were* is correct but the items in the list are incorrectly singular: *The ages, weights, heights and intervals were similar. . ...* *Premedi-cation–induction interval* is better as *interval between premedication and induction* (see Nouns as adjectives, p. 162).

> Thus the magnitude and duration of these rises can be comparable to that following myocardial infarction.

That is singular but refers to *magnitude and duration*; the plural *those* must be used (see also COMPARABLE and FOLLOWING). The *rises* were of the concentrations of enzymes in the plasma; *increases* would be better. It is permissible but not necessary to follow a pair of nouns with a singular verb if the pairing forms a unified concept or implies some other type of closeness: *The art and science of surgery is taught. . ...*

Collective nouns

> . . .and since then a total of 5071 operations have been performed. . .

The subject of *have been* is the singular collective noun *total. 5071 oper-ations have been* but *a total of 5071 operations has been.*

> . . .none of the group developed a fistula and their hospital stay was considerably shorter

NONE (see above) and *group* (a collective noun) are singular and cannot have an attribute (hospital stay) referred to by *their,* which is a plural possessive pronoun. Correct would be: *. . .none of the patients in the group developed a fistula and their hospital stays were* [note plurals] *considerably shorter. Stays in hospital* is better than *hospital stays* (see Nouns as adjectives, p. 162).

The word *number* can take either singular or plural.

> A number of simple texts and papers have been prepared. . .

> Since 1943 the number of aminoglycosides has grown steadily. . .

> Six hundred words are the absolute maximum. . .

In the first example, *number* has plural force; in the second, the amino-glycosides are considered as a unit and the verb is correctly singular (and *increased* is better than *grown*; the microorganisms are grown to produce the antibiotics). The unitary idea (p. 108) requires *is* in the third example, where *number* is implicit after maximum, and where *the maximum* can only be singular: inverting the sentence to *The absolute maximum are 600 words. . .* makes this clear.

> . . . a large percentage of the sport's commentators is called Brian . . .

Percentage is treated the same as *number*: singular as a percentage of a whole (*Fifty per cent of the drug is excreted*) ; plural as a percentage of a number of items (or commentators).

BACTERIA, DATA, CRITERIA

All are plurals: bacteria of bacterium, criteria of criterion, data of datum. Datum is rarely used, and it is likely that data will become a singular noun eventually (p. 56) if only because of its widespread use in computing – not the most literate of subjects. The singular–plural distinctions of the other two words are more important. In an outbreak of legionnaires' disease *The bacteria was found in. . .* should have been either *The bacterium was found in. . .* (if the sense was of the organism identified) or *The bacteria were found in. . ..* Media is also plural, though the word is less common in medical writing, except when referring to tissue culture or microbiological media. In describing methods, remember that it is *The medium* [not media] *was changed every two days.*

> The media has its lighter side. For many it is fun, despite the reservations.

This was from an article about doctors writing and broadcasting. Media might technically be plural, but *The media have their lighter side. For many they are fun. . .* just isn't right, because the focus is the unity and similarity of all media.

But we are not prepared to abandon data yet. The following example from the *British Medical Journal* is correct. In the third sentence the subject is not data but *transfer of data*, which takes the singular.

> The data from the cards were transferred yearly to computer forms. . .
> These data were processed . . . The accuracy of transfer of data at all
> stages was audited and was satisfactory.

The following examples are incorrect:

This data was collected. . .

The data presented in this paper is derived from. . .

The correct plural of *formula* is *formulae* and of *radius* is *radii.* There are many other similar words, derived from Latin or Greek. The *COD* accepts *formulas* and *radiuses,* and they seem more natural in English. Correctly we should use *granulomata* as the plural of *granuloma* and *carcinomata* of *carcinoma*; mostly we prefer to add a simple -s. The plural of cannula (*COD*) is either cannulae or cannulas: pick one and use it but be consistent (mucosae and so on). Beware entanglement in the more difficult Latin endings: we have seen *calvarium* used as the singular for *calvaria* but *calvaria* (the Latin word for skull) is the real singular and *calvariae* the plural. In the recent negotiations for the consultant contract in the United Kingdom, someone invented the plural *premia* for extra payments, but the plural of *premium* is *premiums.* Similarly, the plural of *forum* is not *fora,* but *forums.*

Other examples

They are asked to protrude their tongue to a maximum.

This construction is awkward: *to a maximum* is clumsy; and the patients did not have just a single tongue between them. *They are asked to protrude their tongues as far as possible* is better, and probably paraphrases what the investigators said to their patients (*stick your tongue out as far as you can*). If you dislike *They. . .their tongues* because it is also true that no one had more than one tongue, try: *They are asked to protrude the tongue. . .* or *Each patient was asked to protrude his or her tongue. . .* (see p. 66).

A patient having a successful primary below knee amputation was in hospital a mean of 59 days, whereas. . .

This was not a particular patient who had a number of hospital admissions; it should be *Patients. . .were.*

The subject *patient* and verb *was* are separated by an adjectival clause *having. . .an amputation.* This is not wrong but is a common source of grammatical errors (see p. 174). The example would be better as *Patients were in hospital for a mean of 59 days if their below-knee amputations were successful, whereas. . ..* Note the hyphenation in below-knee.

The nature of injuries to car occupants in 1000 accidents were analysed.

The subject of *were analysed* is not the plural *injuries* but the singular *nature.* The sentence would be better as *We analysed the injuries sustained by the occupants of cars from 1000 accidents* (see NATURE, Nouns as adjectives, p. 162, Use of the passive voice, Chapter 9).

Tenses

The tense of a verb indicates time, which may be *past, present* or *future* (*we showed, we show, we will show*), and completeness of action, which may be *continuous* or completed (*perfect*). Completeness of action may also be in the past, present or future (continuous: *we were showing, we are showing, we will be showing;* perfect: *we had shown, we have shown, we will have shown*).

Medical writers do not need to make a detailed analysis of tenses to write a standard research report, but there are two general guidelines. First, try to keep things simple by using shorter constructions when there is the choice – *we showed* instead of *we have shown; we hoped to show* instead of *we would have liked to have shown.* Writers are more likely to make grammatical errors when using more complex constructions. Secondly, be consistent.

There are subtle ways of using tenses that can convey important nuances of meaning. These are more likely to be understood universally than the 'padding' constructions discussed in the last chapter. Huth (see Reference books, p. 240) deals succinctly with tense in relation to work published in the past. He suggests that *Smith reported that. . .* (the simple past) indicates an event completed. *Smith has reported. . .* (the present perfect) indicates publication in the recent past and implies 'continuing intellectual importance'. *Smith reports that. . .* (the present tense) attaches to a just-published paper of current importance. We agree that these are useful variants (although not appreciated universally) and add that in passive constructions there is a considerable difference between the finality of *It was shown that. . .* and the more open *It has been shown that. . .*, where the signal that there is more to be shown is just about implicit.

A common fault is jumping back and forth between the past and present:

> Smith showed that a single injection was effective but Brown shows a rate of relapse of 30% unless the injection is repeated.

> The pilot tube was attached to the airway by a T-connector so the pressure is equilibrated with the airway pressure.

Tense should be *past* throughout both examples: ... *Brown showed* ... *the injection was*. . .; . . .*the pressure was*. . ..

The usual convention is for the Methods and Results sections of medical papers to be written in the past tense. An exception is a paper containing the first description of a particular method, when the writers may prefer the present tense, which instructs rather than informs:

> The bands are placed around the wrists and ankles, and connected by screened, low capacitance wires.

Figure legends (or captions) are written in the present tense and are the only part of a scientific paper where journals may allow a more terse, telegraphic style: *Dotted line is line of best fit* instead of *The dotted line indicates the line of best fit*.

The Introduction is usually written in the past tense, though this may sometimes not be appropriate throughout. The tense in the Discussion will vary more than elsewhere but must be consistent with the rest of the paper: when referring to another section of the paper, write in the tense you used in that section.

11
Circumlocution, metaphor and cliché

Circumlocution

Do not use lengthy phrases and definitions instead of single words. It is worth asking someone to check over your writing; people unfamiliar with the subject matter of a paper are more likely to detect these circumlocutions. Take this example.

> Oral visual screening . . . has the potential of preventing at least 37000 oral cancer deaths worldwide.

The *COD* definition of *can* is 'potentially capable of': *can prevent* is better here, or, if a little circumspection is needed, *could prevent*. 'Oral visual screening' is *looking in the mouth*.

With some circumlocutions, the fault is not that a particular word has been expanded to its definition, but that the message can be expressed more succinctly. The ability to do this is especially useful when there is a word limit – for instance when submitting abstracts.

> . . . the range of paediatric patients suitable for ventilation . . .

> . . . following open heart surgery in paediatric patients.

Paediatric patients are *children*. Write *neonates, infants* or *older children*, if these are what you are referring to; otherwise *children* is the inclusive term.

> . . . to determine the magnitude of the change in plasma potassium . . .

To determine the magnitude is *to quantify* or *to measure*.

> This comprises of increased blood pressure and pulse amplitude in the upper extremity and decreased blood pressure and pulse amplitude in the legs.

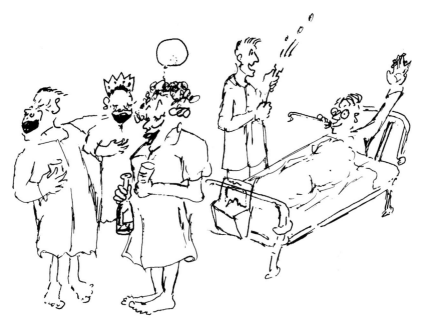

. . . many of our patients remain in hospital for too great a time.

This should be *blood pressure in the arm*; the *upper extremity* can include the shoulder. There is also unnecessary repetition of *blood pressure* and *pulse amplitude* and an incorrect usage – COMPRISES (of).

The actual reason for. . .can only be hypothesized . . .

We can only guess . . . (see HYPOTHESIS, p. 66)

. . . insufficient inpatient accommodation . . .

. . . not enough beds . . .

. . . many of our patients remain in hospital for too great a time . . .

For too great a time means for too long.

. . . the durations of these procedures allowed time to . . .

. . . the procedures were long enough for . . .

. . . due to the brevity of the third stage of labour in most of the patients . . .

. . . because the third stage of labour was usually short . . .

> She was unable to take anything by mouth, including fluids, without choking.

This means *Eating or drinking made her choke.* Using medical terminology: *she had absolute dysphagia.*

> There is not a simple test to predict difficulty . . .

This is an inelegant way of writing *there is no simple test . . .*

> This study is in conformity with previous studies.

> Our findings are at variance with several reports . . .

This form of wording is common in the discussion sections of research papers. It means that the findings do (or do not) agree, confirm or support previous work: *supports* is better than 'in conformity with'; *do not support* is better than 'are at variance with'. The second example is better phrasing, because it is *the findings* of the study, not the study itself, that agree or not with previous findings. Beware too much value judgement on others' work: they will take a different view.

> Patients were asked at this time to indicate to the nurse whether discomfort had been experienced or not.

At this time is *then*. Patients probably *told* the nurse rather than *indicating to* the nurse. They were probably asked whether they had *been in pain* or *been uncomfortable* rather than whether they had *experienced discomfort*. *The nurse then asked the patients whether they had been uncomfortable* is neater.

> The mixed expired concentration can be determined by analysis of a mixed expired sample, or by calculation.

Replace *by analysis of a mixed expired sample* with *by direct measurement.*

> . . . noted a rapid fall to occur during the first trimester to a level which did not change significantly during the remainder of the pregnancy . . .

When writing of the measurement of substances, refer to *increases* and *decreases* rather than *rises* and *falls*, and to *concentrations* rather than *levels*: *there was a rapid decrease during the first trimester to a lower, stable concentration* (see p. 71).

> . . . and the plasma concentration was then manipulated in an upward direction.

Manipulated in an upward direction is *increased*.

> One drawback is the noise [during inflation] –a noise which is similar in character and intensity to that of a suction catheter in operation.

Noise can have only character, intensity and pitch: it has no other attributes. A suction catheter is unlikely to make any noise unless it is 'in operation'. Even then, it is the flow of air produced by the whole suction apparatus that makes the noise. If the writer had been in discussion with a colleague he would probably have said, 'One problem is that it sounds like suction', and something similar to this would have been better in the written report.

> . . . uselessness of the knee joint may make amputation. . .preferable.

The example reads better: *a useless knee joint may make amputation preferable*. ('Detection of pulselessness' has been written for *lack of pulse*.)

> . . . in a concentrated period of time.

Subjectively, time may pass more or less quickly. It cannot be concentrated. The writer meant *over a short period*. *Period* can often be omitted: *for a period of one week* is *for one week*; *for a period lasting two or three months* is *for two or three months*. Similarly, *period of the experiment* usually means just *experiment*.

> It is rapid to perform, the average scan time being five minutes . . .

An immediate improvement is *It is quick*, . . . but the sense is given by the simpler *The average time for a scan is only five minutes* or *A scan takes only about five minutes*.

> The broad indication for invasive measurements can be restated: when the availability of hemodynamic descriptors complement the etiologic and functional diagnosis, define the likely temporal progression of the changing pathophysiology, and modify or may modify the therapeutic approach to management.

The spelling and word formation (*hemodynamic* and *etiologic*) give away the American origin of this example, one of the few in this book. With certain exceptions, notably the *New England Journal of Medicine*, American medical journals contain too many words. Re-restated: . . .*when the hemodynamic measurements complement the clinical diagnosis, indicate the likely prognosis, and are useful in the treatment.*

Short words are not always best (see p. 105).

> Sex involves syngamy, which doubles the amount of DNA in a cell, and meiosis, which halves it.

Sexual reproduction involves syngamy; sex is altogether different.

MADE/MAKE (a particular circumlocution)

> These authors made the suggestion that . . .

> The desire to make contributions . . .

This common construction can usually be replaced by a single verb (*authors suggested . . ., desire to contribute . . .*).

Used in this way, *to make* emphasizes what comes next. *From the evidence, we can make a suggestion: . . .* is more emphatic than *From the evidence, we suggest. . . .* If emphasis is not required, avoid the superfluous *make, made* or *making.*

Metaphor and cliché

Detailed discussion of figures of speech (such as metaphor, simile, oxymoron) are beyond the scope of this book. In general, they should be avoided, mainly because readers may misinterpret them – particularly if English is not their first language. Simple *metaphors* are often used by medical writers.

Metaphor (COD) is the application of name or descriptive term to an object or action to which it is imaginatively but not literally applicable. Metaphor is sometimes useful to aid understanding of a difficult idea, but otherwise should not be used in scientific papers.

A fashionable metaphorical expression is *in depth. The damaged cars were examined in depth* (see p. 165) means that the cars were examined *in detail,* or *thoroughly. An in-depth review* is a common replacement for *a thorough review.*

> . . . and this deficiency may play a role in the genesis of postoperative deep vein thrombosis.

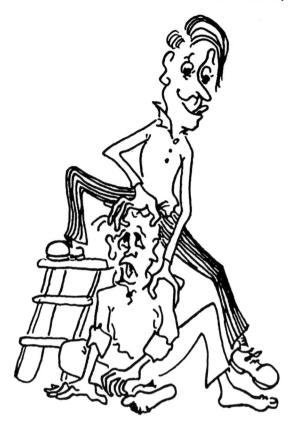

You shouldn't tread on people's toes by going over their heads.

An actor *may play a role* (see p. 89); a deficiency *may be a factor. Formation* is better than *genesis.* The example is better rewritten: *. . . and this deficiency may make postoperative deep vein thrombosis more likely.*

Metaphors may cause unintended hilarity. My wife told me that while lecturing to medical students one day she had inadvertently said (of referring a GP's patients from her own hospital department to another department): 'You shouldn't tread on peoples' toes by going over their heads.' None of the students seemed to notice. (This is an example of a *mixed metaphor.* Another example was the Union official, incensed at large pay rises awarded to directors of privatized utilities, who spoke of them 'having their snouts in the gravy train'.)

Many expressions are so common that they are no longer thought of as metaphors. They are *dead metaphors* and are easily reawakened, sometimes with ludicrous results. When applied to NHS Trusts, '[Many] of them were managing to keep their heads above water', though not a metaphor of great imagination, conveys the idea of *coping reasonably well*. As a quotation (which it is) from the National Association of Head Teachers, it brings a different picture to mind.

Here are two more:

> The Sports Council is responsible for collecting the samples [of urine] and making sure the procedures are watertight.

> [They are] negotiating contracts that hammer British Coal into the ground.

Mental images of urine spurting from specimen tubes and lumps of coal being pushed back under the earth interfere with the intended messages.

This is from an article warning about the need to take statutory form E111 when going on holiday from the UK to a European Community country.

> Millions of holidaymakers are leaving themselves vulnerable to unnecessary headaches in recovering medical costs they are entitled to as a UK resident . . .

One hopes that the E111 covers more than just headaches.

> The orthopaedic department cannot cope with the volume of fractures it has to see. A spokesman said, 'They have reached breaking point.'

Indeed they have.

Another danger of metaphors is that they can become clichés. Metaphors are intended to enliven writing; clichés, because they are overused, deaden it. There is no strict definition of cliché; nor is there a list in which to check whether a chosen metaphor has degenerated to cliché. As the *Longman's Guide to English Usage* (currently out of print) pointed out, many clichés are verbiage, expressions that are a substitute for independent thinking and that have 'lost . . . force and freshness because of overuse'.

> But at the end of the day there may be a much better service for patients, as well as better training for juniors.

But the result may be . . .

> And at the end of the day [women] own less than 1% of the world's property.

Women don't own any more than 1% of the property early in the morning or in the middle of the night; the sentence is better, and its initial *and* is more effective, without the phrase.

A good example of *cliché* in this world of high-technology medicine (itself a cliché) is *state-of-the-art* to mean *the latest, the most advanced*. Never use it. Philip Howard, in *Winged words*,[37] described a British Telecom slogan 'We're responsible for a host of other state-of-the-art innovations' as using language like breaking wind. An equally ripe flatus is *quantum leap*, which has the double disadvantage of being gibberish and overused.

Gold standard is a much favoured cliché in medical writing. Usually it means no more than 'the best method we have at the moment', which is better expressed explicitly as *current best practice*.

> [The m]ain outcome measure [was p]erformance of the diagnostic test against a gold standard consisting of either a 48 hour measurement of troponin T concentration or screening for myocardial infarction according to the World Health Organization's criteria.

Two gold standards is simply ridiculous: the economic measure was the value of gold; the value altered but not the metal. Writing of *a* gold standard is also rather silly: it was *the* gold standard; that was its point. In this example, *gold* can be omitted: *a standard* will do.

> [The m]ain outcome measures [were t]he sensitivity, specificity, precision ("positive predictive value"), and accuracy. . . determined by comparison with a hand search of all articles (the "gold standard") . . .

Perhaps the authors were embarrassed about gold standard, and so cloaked it in inverted commas. Better simply to have said that a hand search was the best method, and from then on to have compared with 'the hand search'. The inverted commas around *positive predictive value* are unnecessary and confusing. They suggest the authors invented or borrowed the term (as they did gold standard), but positive predictive value is a defined statistic, and the intention here is to state the index by which precision was measured.

If you use metaphors in your writing keep them simple and use them sparingly. The advice in most books on usage is to use your judgement.

Perhaps the best general advice is not to write what you find annoying or would ridicule in others' writing. Avoid metaphors heard in committee meetings and used by politicians. Too many of us have to write to tight deadlines (a metaphor taken from a line beyond which prisoners were liable to be shot), but taking the time to ask a colleague to criticize your writing (see p. 29) is especially effective for spotting inappropriate metaphors.

Metaphors are especially common in managerial communications: at the coal-face, levelling the playing field and moving the goalposts; ear-marking, ring-fencing and top-slicing. Understand that *human resource downsizing* means *giving people the sack* and *downward cost adjustment* means *cuts* and you will be less impressed by the language (also see euphemism). Doctors are not innocent: *patients with positive treatment outcomes* are *patients who do well* (see p. 16).

12
Word order and pronouns

Nouns, adjectives and prepositions do not change their endings in English to indicate how they relate to each other. Words can be stressed in speech, but although underlining and italics will indicate stress in writing they are devices to use sparingly. Some journals will not accept italicized emphases. In written English, meaning is determined first by the positions, or presumed positions, of words, phrases and clauses, and second by the punctuation between them.

Consider this simple example.

The policy was changed after a near clinical disaster.

Readers expect *near* to qualify the word next to it, *clinical*. Although it takes only a moment to realize that the sense is of *a clinical near-disaster* and not of *a disaster that was nearly clinical*, the expression is a jolt to the flow of understanding. The example is better as *The policy was changed after there was nearly a clinical disaster.*

Sometimes the interpreted meaning may be far from the intended one, as in this letter from a firm of solicitors to a general practice:

We feel it can only improve our service to clients, particularly as [many] of our personal injury/domestic violence clients seek our assistance after visiting your health centre.

Note the 'lazy slash', which is better replaced with *and*: see p. 178.

Missing words

Words are often left out but their position is assumed and understood by readers as if they were there:

> The dose of morphine is 10 mg, and of heroin is 5 mg.

The words *the dose* are understood in the second part of this sentence: . . ., *and the dose of heroin is 5 mg*. The grammatical term is *ellipsis*.

Ambiguity can occur if writers do not consider the possible misinterpretations that can arise because of ellipsis.

> Adverse reactions to drugs and anaesthetists.

This can be misinterpreted by mischievously assuming the ellipsis of *to*: *Adverse reactions to drugs and* [to] *anaesthetists*. Reversing the example, the title of an editorial, avoids ambiguity: *Anaesthetists and adverse reactions to drugs*.

Putting the simpler construction first (the single word *anaesthetists*) and the less simple construction second (*adverse reactions to drugs*) prevents words from the longer group governing the shorter.

> Although oral examinations are less objective they can be made more reliable by careful structuring and training of examiners.

There is ellipsis of *of the examiners* after *structuring*, and there may be ellipsis of *careful* before *training*. But at first reading, that there is no *by* before *training* gives the sense that it is the examiners who need structuring.

Ellipsis of small words is a common source of ambiguity. Even the occasional omission of the definite or indefinite articles (*the, a, an*) can cause a surprising amount of confusion because they have such strong effects on the attached noun. Some medical writers mistakenly pare away almost all the articles in the cause of brevity (usually leaving in their text all sorts of other superfluities) or in search of spurious style. There is a difference between useful editing and purposeless defleshing. Text deprived of most of the articles is difficult to interpret and actually appears more turgid than its longer version with these vital parts of speech intact. How to use definite and indefinite articles properly is a specific problem for some writers whose first language is not English.

Nouns as adjectives

Nouns can act as adjectives. *The biochemistry department* is more common usage than *the department of biochemistry*. Some examples have been discussed in previous sections: *liver metastases, stomach cancer* and *plasma concentration* are acceptable for *metastases in the liver, cancer of the stomach* and *concentration in the plasma*. Some authorities will not accept the use of nouns as adjectives at all, though as we have expressions in English such as *railway station, door handle, county council* and *customs officer*, this condemnation is excessive. Gowers comments:

> the constant use of such phrases is usually a sign of unclear thinking. . . a phrase consisting of more than two words should be treated with suspicion, and things tend to get even more awkward if the phrase includes an adjective as well as a number of nouns; it is not always obvious on first reading which noun the adjective qualifies, and tiresome problems of hyphenation arise.

Medical writing is littered with these strings, or stacks, of noun qualifiers or modifiers. Where they are ambiguous it can be impossible for a sub-editor to decide what the writer intended. This leads to mistakes if the sub takes a leap in the dark, and the alternative is tedious, time-consuming queries to the writer.

> . . . three day unit sessions . . .

Is this *three sessions in the day unit* or *unitary sessions of three days*? The ambiguity could be avoided by using a hyphen, *three day-unit sessions*, but writing *three sessions in the day unit* is clearer.

> . . . a series of fixed duration sequential constant rate infusions . . .

Hyphens improve understanding (*fixed-duration sequential constant-rate infusions*) but not the writing. Rearranged as *sequential infusions of constant rate and fixed duration* it is immediately obvious which adjective is qualifying which noun. With better style, one can then see that *a series of* is superfluous, as something that is sequential must be a series.

> Another aspect of crevicular fluid biochemical profile complexity . . .

This is the *complexity of the biochemical profile of crevicular fluid*.

> The growth factor involvement in this regeneration process has been rather extensively studied.

Here the stacked modifier *growth factor* introduces an ambiguity common in this type of construction. The *involvement* is actually of *several* growth factors not the singular growth factor, but the word order cannot convey this important fact. *The involvement of growth factors . . .* removes the ambiguity.

> At present, health care cost containment remains a national priority . . .

As in the previous example *of* makes the meaning clearer: *containment of the cost of health care.* The whole example is a euphemism for *we have to see how we can provide a medical service as cheaply as possible.*

> Smoke inhalation injury is a major factor in fire victim mortality.

There is no need here to write *mortality* for *death* (see FATALITY). Some writers might prefer the phrase *smoke inhalation injury* to *injury from inhalation of smoke* for its convenience and as a definition of the specific condition, but in the example *injury* is superfluous: *Inhalation of smoke is an important factor in deaths after fires* (see MAJOR).

> By using a series of delay times 16 msec apart . . .

Delay describes *times* but a delay is a time so *times* is superfluous. A delay is *a time between events,* so it is not correct to describe delays as *being apart.* Try: *By using a series of delays, each of 16ms. . . .* The not uncommon *period of time* (see p. 51) is a similar tautology.

> Insulin sensitivity is increased among people who consume on average one to three alcohol containing drinks a day.
>
> The coefficients for alcohol from beer, wine, and spirits were not significantly different from each other or from the coefficient among the remaining studies that provided either ethanol or non-specific alcohol containing beverages
>
> Patients abstained from alcohol and caffeine containing drinks for 24 hours before the study.

It is the drinks that contain alcohol, not the alcohol that contains the drinks, so it is odd that writers seem to prefer the clumsier construction. The phrase *alcohol and caffeine containing drinks* is better as *drinks containing alcohol or caffeine,* although many subeditors would simply 'hang' a hyphen after *alcohol* and hyphenate *caffeine-containing.* To *abstain* is (*COD*) to restrain oneself from, not the right sense for the 24 hours before a study. *Don't drink alcohol, coffee or tea for the 24 hours before the study* is probably what the patients were told. *Alcohol* (*COD*) can also be any liquor that contains it, so similar phrasing will suffice in the writing as in the instruction.

The second example is better as: 'that provided beverages containing either ethanol or non-specific alcohol'.

> A car occupant ejection study found that rear-seat ejection was hazardous.

> The probability of occupant ejection is increased with vehicle rollovers.

The first of these examples means *it is dangerous to be thrown from the rear seat of a car*. It does not mean that occupants will be injured if the rear seat is ejected from the vehicle, which is what is written. The second means that *people are more likely to be thrown out if a vehicle rolls over*.

This is from the same paper:

> Current model cars that were damaged severely enough to be towed away from the accident scene were investigated in depth.

Current model cars should be *cars of a current model* unless they were children's toys; *accident scene* should be *scene of the accident* but is superfluous. There is no need to write the metaphorical *in depth, thoroughly* is the correct word (see p. 156). An accident is *investigated* but a damaged car is *inspected* or *examined*: *Cars of a current model that were so badly damaged that they had to be towed away were inspected thoroughly.*

Even better is to reverse the sentence and use the passive in a different way (p. 139), which avoids the long separation between the subject *cars* and its verb *were inspected*. This separation is not incorrect, but it is awkward. Rewritten: *A thorough inspection was made of cars of a current model that were so badly damaged they had to be towed away.*

> These substances reduce nervous activity in laboratory conditions and these findings have been confirmed in patient studies.

The writers meant that the findings had been confirmed in studies of patients, not in studies that were careful and painstaking. A scientific study must be done with careful, precise, thought. So must the writing when the study is reported.

> Because only K^+ evoked noradrenaline release is extracellular Ca^{2+} dependent our data suggest block of Ca^{2+} channels.

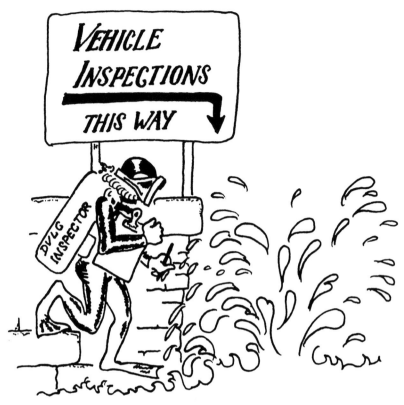

Current model cars . . . were investigated in depth.

The strings of modifiers create a number of false starts when reading this sentence. *Evoked* is read first as a verb (*It was only potassium that evoked the release of noradrenaline*), but that analysis is incorrect – which readers realize when they reach *is*. Sentences that mislead readers on first reading are termed *garden path sentences*, because they 'lead . . ."up the garden path" to an incorrect analysis'. Re-analysis makes the potassium cause release of the noradrenaline (a hyphen makes this clear: K^+-evoked noradrenaline release). It then seems that the release of noradrenaline is extracellular (a reasonable idea), until reading the next word suggests that the release *is* extracellular calcium. (Note that K^+ and Ca^{2+} are abbreviations (see p. 188) for the charged ion; there is no need to write K^+ *ion*, K^+ means potassium ion.) Another re-analysis is needed: the release is *dependent on* extracellular calcium. Rewriting, with a single hyphen, makes the sentence clear at first reading: *We suggest the mechanism is by block of Ca^{2+} channels, because only K^+-evoked release of noradrenaline is dependent on extracellular Ca^{2+}.*

In our opinion, to realize the problems created by strings of unfamiliar modifiers is the simplest single way to improve medical writing. (And not just medical writing: did *The Guardian* really mean to describe a member of a pop group as a 'fake tan-loving singer'?) Writers should also remember that judicious punctuation of the strings helps the editor and readers to sort out what is meant. Sometimes the difficulty of placing sensible punctuation will show that all is not well. Somehow we doubt if this example from an advert in the medical press could have been made less dubious or offensive by punctuation: 'Wanted: brown fat research assistant.'

Adverbs and verbs

Adverbs qualify verbs, adjectives or other adverbs. To prevent ambiguity, adverbs should usually be near the words they qualify.

It is the position of the adverb that causes the argument about the split infinitive. Writers who know of no other rules of grammar have often heard of two: that the split infinitive is wrong and that a sentence should never end with a preposition. Most grammarians agree that neither rule is absolute. There are many principles of grammar that are far more important, and it is odd that these two, particularly the split infinitive, are so well known.

The infinitive is the form *to be, to study,* or *to calculate.* The rule about the split infinitive holds that nothing should come between *to* and the so-called bare infinitive: thus *to carefully study* would be wrong. The split infinitive is still debated by grammarians but Gowers' advice is good for medical writers: 'It is also a bad rule, which many people (including good writers) reject. It increases the difficulty of writing clearly and makes for ambiguity by inducing writers to place adverbs in unnatural and even misleading places.' It goes on, however: 'Opposition to the split infinitive remains powerful. It is therefore wiser to avoid splitting your infinitives. There is nearly always an easy and natural way for doing so.'

The aim of this book is to make medical articles more readable, not grammatically correct for grammar's sake. The best test for medical writers is does splitting an infinitive make the writing clumsy, alter the sense or introduce ambiguity? Technically, infinitives include not just *to study* but forms like the past infinitive *to have studied,* the present continuous infinitive *to be studying*, or the past continuous infinitive *to have been studying*. The same test applies to inserting words into these forms.

The same principles apply to putting an adverb between the subject and the verb. Which is correct: *he ran quickly* or *he quickly ran?* In speech, the stressed syllable (indicated by a short vertical dash, for example *commu'nicate*) informs that *he ran quick'ly*, implying that he ran quickly *not slowly*. Interposing the adverb gives *he quickly ran'*, implying he ran *instead of walking*. In correct written English, the adverb can be before or after the verb. The correct position should be decided on each occasion by thinking carefully about ease, sense and ambiguity.

Adverbs of frequency sit comfortably between subject and verb: *we always injected . . .*; *melanomas sometimes regress. . . .* Consider this example from the *British Medical Journal*:

> Patients with this condition who present as abdominal emergencies are frequently reported.

The stress is on the last word of the sentence *reported* (the same as *he quickly ran'*) and the implication is that patients are likely to be reported if they present as abdominal emergencies. This is exactly what the writers meant with no suggestion that this reporting is frequent; *. . . are reported frequently* puts the emphasis on *frequently* and implies that the journals are inundated by reports.

> . . . an infusion exponentially decreasing with time . . .

The mode of decrease is being described: *a rate of infusion decreasing exponentially with time* is better. As quoted, the phrase contrasts with a rate of infusion exponentially *increasing* with time.

> . . . insufficient attention has previously been paid [to technique] . . .

If needed at all (see p. 72), *previously* should precede the main clause: *. . . previously, insufficient attention has been paid [to technique]. . . .*

> . . . disproved by X and Y who separately blocked with drugs the local innervation of the blood vessels and the sweat glands . . .

This is ambiguous: does *separately* refer to X and Y, or to the blocking of the innervation? A better phrasing is *. . . who blocked the local innervation . . . separately with drugs*, but the cause of the problem is poor choice of word: *separately* here means *selectively* and writing *selectively* avoids the ambiguity.

> Humans with damage to the amygdala have difficulty perceiving fear on someone's face and do not learn normally to identify stimuli that signal danger.

The writer, perhaps wary of splitting the infinitive, has introduced an ambiguity that arises because normally can mean either *in the usual manner* or *as a rule*. Consequently, we don't know whether damage to the amygdala prevents normal learning (the intended meaning) or means that usually the patients do not learn (unintended). Splitting the infinitive (*to normally identify*) is unambiguous but clumsy. Better is *to identify normally stimuli*. . . . It is not easy to explain why, but the best style is to be more specific about stimuli, and insert the article: . . . *to identify normally the stimuli that signal danger.*

This is an illustration of how style in English is a feel for language, for what feels and sounds right. Rules and guidance help; seek and destroy missions on *It has been noted that* are worthwhile, but in the end there is no substitute for practice and familiarity.

> Traditionally surgical procedures on the knee joint have been performed through arthrotomy incisions.

The position of *traditionally* makes it qualify *surgical procedures*. Actually it is qualifying *performed*. Try: . . . *have been performed traditionally through.* . . . A neater alternative is to insert a comma: *Traditionally, surgical procedures.* . . .

Sentences beginning with adverbs are sometimes better rewritten:

> Histologically, they fall into two distinct groups . . .

They form two distinct histological groups is better. Literal verbs are better in medical writing than figurative verbs: *form* is better than *fall into* (see p. 70).

A troublesome word: ONLY

Only, depending on its position, can change the meaning of a sentence completely.

1 Only the operation can relieve the condition [not drugs].
2 The only operation can relieve the condition [there are no other operations].
3 The operation only can relieve the condition [ambiguous, could be (1) or (4)].

4 The operation can only relieve the condition [it cannot cure it].

5 The operation can relieve only the condition [not for example, the social consequences]

6 The operation can relieve the only condition [there are no other conditions].

7 The operation can relieve the condition only [could be (4) or (5)].

There is less likelihood of ambiguity when *only* is close to the word it qualifies but even the best of writers make mistakes with *only*:

> . . . those who inherit this gene from one parent only enjoy a significant degree of protection against subtertain [falciparum] malaria.

At first reading, *only* is taken to qualify *enjoy*, but it should qualify *one parent*: . . . *those who inherit this gene from only one parent enjoy*. . . . As the writer of this example was Sir Peter Medawar, one of the most distinguished and effective medical communicators ever, we shall remain humble.

In the following example, the misplaced word is *solely* rather than *only*:

> The fact that histamine release can be related to particular surgical events further emphasises that the anaesthetic agent may not solely be involved with adverse reactions.

The writers wanted to stress that factors other than the anaesthetic agent can be responsible for adverse reactions. This is not clear from their writing, which suggests that the anaesthetic may be implicated in something other than adverse reactions. The faults are the misplacement of *solely* and the imprecise use of *involve* (see INVOLVED, p. 112). No matter where *solely* (or *only*) is placed, the sentence remains awkward because it is the wrong way round. Try: *Anaesthetic agents are not the only cause of adverse reactions, particular surgical events can also cause the release of histamine.*

Pronouns and nouns

The mouse in Lewis Carroll's *Alice's Adventures Through the Looking Glass* was telling a story.

> 'I proceed. "Edwin and Morcar . . . and even Stigand, the patriotic archbishop of Canterbury, found it advisable – "'

'Found *what*?' said the duck.

'Found *it*,' the mouse replied rather crossly: 'of course you know what "it" means.'

'I know what "it" means well enough, when *I* find a thing,' said the duck: 'it's generally a frog or a worm. The question is, what did the archbishop find?'

Make sure that *it, they* or other pronouns refer unambiguously to their correct nouns. Mistakes are most likely when a pronoun refers to a noun in a previous sentence – sometimes even in a previous paragraph. If in doubt, repeat the antecedent noun.

> In other words, our political masters find doctors obstructive and difficult because they subscribe to a system of ethics and standards over which they have no managerial control.

To what do the two *theys* refer? The context made it clear that doctors have the ethics, and the politicians want control, but it is better to be explicit by repeating the nouns. *In other words, our political masters find doctors obstructive and difficult because doctors subscribe to a system of ethics and standards over which politicians have no managerial control.*

Be careful also with relative pronouns (see WHICH, p. 132), and possessive pronouns (*its, their*):

> [Of angiography] . . . there have been few reports of its use in paediatric practice with its different spectrum of pathology.

The first *its* refers to angiography, the second to paediatric practice. Try . . . *there have been few reports of its use in paediatric practice, in which there is . . .,* but there are other improvements.

Children or *by paediatricians* would probably be better than *in paediatric practice*, and *disease* better than *pathology* (see also SPECTRUM, p. 91). Presumably, the writers are pointing out that children differ from adults, and this is better stated explicitly unless the contrast has already been made. Rewritten, the example reads: . . . *there are few reports of its use in children, who have different diseases from adults.*

> Smith *et al.* repeated the study of Brown *et al.* These workers used a different staining technique . . .

Many writers are wary of repeating the same words in the same sentence, or sometimes in the same paragraph or on the same page. It is better to write the names explicitly, no matter how many times this is necessary, than to leave any confusion in the minds of readers over whether *These workers* refers to Smith's or Brown's group. The same applies to the device of writing *This latter study*; repeating the names is clearer (see LATTER, p. 136).

13
Punctuation

Medical writers tend to write long sentences in which one subordinate clause comes after another, sometimes with no punctuation at all. Readers may have to read a sentence two or three times to get the sense. Short sentences are more likely to be clear and less likely to cause ambiguity. This chapter deals with the basic ideas of punctuation. In Chapter 14, there is a more general discussion of the construction of sentences. (For the use of apostrophes, see p. 38.)

Punctuation has been having a much better than customary press after the runaway success of Lynne Truss's book, *Eats, Shoots and Leaves* (see Books to read, p. 242). Anyone who has read that book can regard this chapter as revision.

Full stops and a few commas should suffice. (Full stops are *periods* to North Americans, and *full points* to editors.) Use colons and semi-colons only if you know how. Only a full stop, not a colon, is followed by a capital letter: the text following a colon is part of the same sentence.

Some rules of punctuation are:

- a semi-colon is almost a full stop;
- use a colon to introduce a list;
- separate the items on a list by commas not semi-colons (unless the items could themselves be sentences or have commas within them);
- if you use commas to mark a parenthesis, like this, you must pair them just as you would always close a bracket;
- never separate a subject from its verb by a single punctuation mark.

It is sometimes helpful when checking punctuation to read a doubtful passage aloud, exaggerating the pauses; this may show where the punctuation is incorrect or lacking, or where meaning has been altered or made ambiguous by punctuation. A simple rule is that if readers have to read a sentence twice it is a bad sentence.

One sometimes encounters medical books, often the latest of several editions by a senior authority, that have impeccable style and minimal punctuation. To modern readers, these have a strange look and in places are difficult to read. It used to be a mark of style in literature of any kind to restrain punctuation, especially the comma. We do not advocate unbridled punctuation, but it can ease the ingestion of difficult medical writing to err on the side of slightly too many commas. What follows shows where commas should not intrude.

Commas between subject and verb

There should never be a single comma between subject and verb. There are signs that this mistake is a new focus of infection in medical writing. No one would write *The drug, caused nausea,* but that is the effect of this mistake. It is common when writers interpose long strings of words between subject and verb.

> Analysis of the results obtained after one minute, indicates that. . .

> Awareness and recall during anaesthesia and surgery, have been reported . . .

> An example of this, is the treatment of pain arising from the cervical spine.

> Abstracts which are not readable in English, will regrettably be returned without review.

The commas should be omitted.

> Upper limb paralysis following the use of a tourniquet to establish a bloodless field, was formerly a well known complication . . .

Either delete the comma, or add one after *paralysis.* It is acceptable to have a pair of commas between subject and verb although too many commas make the style jerky and distracting.

There are other faults in the example. *Upper limb paralysis* would be better as *paralysis of the upper limb* (see Nouns as adjectives, p. 162). *Used to be* is more elegant than *was formerly. After* is better than *following.*

> The clinical decision – that is the action recommended when reporting on the photograph – even though some detail may not have been recorded, agreed with direct assessment by the ophthalmologist in *x*% of cases.

This is a complicated sentence in which there are two parentheses. The first is enclosed by dashes and qualifies *the clinical decision*; the second is between the second dash and the comma and qualifies *the reporting of the photograph*. That comma splits subject and verb: *decision* and *agreed*.

The second parenthesis qualifies the first, so both parentheses should be within the dashes: *The clinical decision – that is the action recommended when reporting on the photograph, even though some detail may not have been recorded – agreed with direct assessment by the ophthalmologist in x% of cases.* The comma within the parenthesis does not split the subject and verb. Some writers use the parenthetic dash too much. A page of text liberally sprinkled with these is likely to be difficult to read because they do not adequately control unruly clauses.

> . . . this option was discussed with, and accepted, by the patient . . .

This comma is not misplaced between a subject and verb but between a verb and a preposition. The option was *discussed with* and *accepted by* the patient. Omitting the parenthesis between the commas produces *this option was discussed with by the patient*. The commas are not necessary. The example would be better as . . . *this option was accepted by the patient after discussion. . . .*

It is easy to get commas wrong, which was the whole point of the title of *Eats, Shoots and Leaves*. A medical journal had appealed for editorial consultants, commenting:

> We have aimed for an international panel of consultants. Perhaps, unsurprisingly, most applicants came from Europe or North America.

A comma has crept in after *perhaps*, pushing *unsurprisingly* parenthetically aside and suggesting the journal did not know where the applicants had come from.

Lists

Items in a list are separated by commas, or by semi-colons if the items contain commas or are themselves sentences. A colon can precede a list.

The last item is usually preceded by *and* (or *or*). Whether the final *and* must be preceded by a comma is a matter of opinion. It is seldom wrong to use one in a simple list, but consider this example.

> Treatment consisted of graded exercises, beta-blockers, avoiding fatty foods(,) and giving up cigarettes.

The comma is optional, though some say you should be consistent and either always have one or never have one. Some authorities maintain that the final comma is a way of putting extra stress on the last item, and that this purpose is lost if the comma is always there. A more certain way of stressing the last item is to use a dash: . . . *beta-blockers, avoiding fatty foods – and giving up cigarettes.* Dashes, as we have said, should be used sparingly.

> Treatment consisted of graded exercises, beta-blockers, avoiding fatty foods, and cigarettes.

A comma is now wrong, because there is an understood *avoiding* before *cigarettes*: treatment includes *avoiding fatty foods and avoiding cigarettes* (see ellipsis, p. 162). A comma makes *cigarettes* part of the treatment.

> Treatment consisted of graded exercises, beta-blockers, avoiding fatty foods and giving up cigarettes, which have an importance most patients find easy to ignore.

This is ambiguous if your habit is never to insert a comma before the final *and*: is it *cigarettes* that have the importance (in the causation) or is it *the avoiding of fatty foods and the giving up of cigarettes* that have an importance (in the treatment)? Putting , *and* removes the ambiguity; it must now be cigarettes that have the importance. Note that *giving up cigarettes* is singular and, if the final construction were *which has an importance most patients find easy to ignore*, it would refer unambiguously to it.

> The principal aims are rapid acquisition of strength, minimal tissue damage with minimal inflammation and a good scar.

There should be a comma after *inflammation* to indicate that *inflammation* is included with *tissue damage* but that *the scar* is a separate item in the list.

> It is ironic that the two met for the first time in Stockholm to receive their prizes; Golgi's speech was an attack on neuron theory, Cajal followed with a tactful defense.

The semi-colon should be a colon, introducing a list of two items that could each stand as a sentence and thus need a semi-colon between them. Note the American spelling of defence. (Whatever the vehemence of his attack, Golgi was wrong.)

This next example confusingly mixes commas, dashes and a semi-colon.

> This book successfully shows us at our most elementary – a mass of DNA, gene products, and instincts – and our most sophisticated; intelligent, capable of mature reflection, and cooperating in a joint endeavour to solve life's predicaments.

The second list (of sophisticated things) is separated from its introduction by an incorrect semi-colon. Inserting a dash to restore balance with the first list (of elementary things) leaves *and our most sophisticated* awkwardly marked off as if it is in parentheses. A separating semi-colon is needed after *instincts*. The choice is for dashes or colons to mark the start of each list. The commas within the lists are correct.

> *This book successfully shows us at our most elementary: a mass of DNA, gene products, and instincts; and our most sophisticated: intelligent, capable of mature reflection, and cooperating in a joint endeavour to solve life's predicaments.*

Some lists are complicated:

> We found several problems with this system; the results could be biased by the person asking each patient to describe their pain in this way, asking patients to make repeated observations was time-consuming and could involve several different people – which introduced changes in bias, and finally, a mountain of paper could be generated which was difficult to handle.

A comment made by someone who read this was, 'There is no way to make sense of this rubbish other than by rewriting it.' That is an exaggeration: it may not be clear but the writers have used good, simple words. The metaphor (see p. 156) of *a mountain of paper* is effective; *a large amount of paper* would be weak.

A good way to avoid submitting incomprehensible rubbish to journals is to give an early draft of your paper to someone unconnected with the study. They will not have preconceived ideas of what you think you have written.

The list in the example is: bias of results, repeated observations, and a mountain of paper. The sentence is confusing because it is difficult to separate the items in the list from the phrases and clauses that qualify the items. It could be punctuated as a list with a colon after *system* and a semi-colon after *changes in bias,* but rewriting is better:

> *We found several problems with this system. First, the results could be biased by the particular way that investigators asked the patients to describe pain. Secondly, asking patients to make repeated observations was time-consuming and could involve several different people, which introduced further bias. Lastly, the process generated an unmanageable mountain of paper.*

The lazy slash

A previous example included 'our personal injury/domestic violence clients'. This, what we term 'lazy slash', usually does nothing more than save writing the word *and* or *or.* Here, *our personal injury and domestic violence clients* is better. It is anyway impossible to speak this phrase without adding *and.* Symptoms that commonly occur together are often joined by a slash, as in *pain/numbness,* or by the compound conjunction *and/or,* as in *heartburn and/or nausea.* At least *and/or* can be spoken, but *and/or* is almost always an unnecessary expansion of *and.*

He/she is a common use of the slash. There are better ways of avoiding accusations of sexism (see p. 65).

14

Constructing sentences

Balance

The most important grammatical guide to the construction of sentences is that segments should have equal value. A segment of a sentence may be a phrase or a clause. A phrase is defined as a segment without a finite verb, so a word can be considered a short phrase. Segments are divided by punctuation and joined by conjunctions. The simplest conjunction is *and*.

The word BOTH allows a good illustration of what is meant by segments of equal value.

Ewing's sarcoma occurs both in flat bones and in long bones.

The two phrases that follow *both* (joined by *and*) each contain a preposition (in), an adjective (flat, long) and a noun (bones). The two phrases do not have to be the same length (*in children's growing flat bones* has the same value), but balance is lost if one segment contains a finite verb:

Ewing's sarcoma both occurs in flat bones and in long bones.

Here *both* governs a finite verb (*occurs*) in the first segment (which is now a clause), and the lack of a finite verb in the second segment throws the reader. A balanced sentence is:

Ewing's sarcoma both occurs in flat bones and is common in children.

In this next example, *both* should come after *reduces*. The two balanced segments are in italics.

. . . the addition of cyclizine to morphine both reduces *nausea* and *the need for further antiemetic treatment.*

Again the two segments are in italics:

> Outcomes research presumably both *solves the problem of quality and cost that beset the health care system* and *does so by scientific rather than political means.*

The second *and* joins the equal segments governed by *both*, which are main clauses. The first main clause is complicated, containing a subordinate clause (*quality and cost that beset the health care system*). The *and* within that clause does not have the same weight as the *and* joining the two main clauses, but the meaning of the sentence is clear from the flow of the words, without needing punctuation.

> The big rise [in mumps] has occurred despite repeated warnings to inoculate young people for whom the disease can be particularly painful, and in a small minority of cases, a serious threat to health.

As it reads, with no comma before *for whom*, the warning is to inoculate just those young people in whom mumps will be painful, but the phrase *for whom the disease can be particularly painful* applies to all young people, and a comma is essential. The comma after *painful* should be moved to after *and*: the disease is painful and a threat. *A small minority* is better replaced by a percentage.

Rewritten: *The big rise [in mumps cases] has occurred despite repeated warnings to inoculate young people, for whom the disease can be particularly painful and, in about x%, a serious threat to health.*

In this extract from a travel brochure, expecting *and* to link segments of equal value suggests planes full of weekend insects:

> Our special Saturday flight is on a scheduled seat configuration allowing for greater comfort and flies over the weekend.

The complexity of the grammar of sentences and the likelihood of making grammatical mistakes are lessened by keeping sentences short. In both English literature and scientific writing, long sentences used to be fashionable. They are less so nowadays. Many great living writers of English use long sentences to good effect, but most medical writers are not great writers and it is better to keep sentences simple.

> The appearance of a small or moderate quantity of air in this position may not be appreciated although a greater quantity of intrapleural air

permits further lung retraction revealing the familiar pleural line parallel to the lateral chest wall.

This sentence is too long to have no punctuation. The simplest satisfactory punctuation is one comma after *appreciated* and another after *retraction*. This makes the sentence easier to understand but grammatically incorrect because the construction is then of unequal segments: clause, clause, phrase. Correct punctuation for a single sentence requires a semi-colon after *appreciated*: clause; clause, phrase.

Even when punctuated, the passage is poor style. Writers tend to write good English (good choice of words, correct punctuation) or poor English. It is particularly unusual to see a poor choice of words with correct punctuation. Here, *the appearance of* is superfluous; *amount* is better than *quantity*; *appreciated* should be *noticed* or *recognized*; *a greater quantity of* is *more*; *allows* is better than *permits*; and the lung *collapses*, it does not *retract*.

Rewritten: *A small or moderate amount of air in this position may not be noticed. More intrapleural air allows further collapse, revealing the familiar pleural line. . . .*

A cancellation by the hospital is a tragedy but this can perhaps only be prevented or minimised by introducing day case facilities or by allocating specific beds for elective admissions that cannot be used for emergency cases.

Thirty-seven words without punctuation: readers have no idea of the relative emphasis of the words or of their relation one to another. On first reading, the last clause *that cannot be used for emergency cases*, which should qualify *specific beds*, appears to qualify *elective admissions*. A few words should be changed (a cancelled operation is not a tragedy) but the main improvement comes from punctuation.

Rewritten: *A cancellation by the hospital is inconvenient for the patient. The only way of preventing or minimising this is to introduce facilities for day cases or to allocate specific beds for elective admissions, ensuring these beds are not used for emergency cases.*

Leakage past the tourniquet has been reported by many workers and radiocontrast studies show that this leakage commonly occurs through the venous system although further routes of possible leakage are the interosseous circulation, which will bypass the tourniquet and the failure of a tourniquet to occlude calcified arteries.

The ideas are in the correct order, but the passage is poorly written as well as needing punctuation for balance. The most needed punctuation is a few full stops.

Rewritten: *Many workers have reported leakage past tourniquets. Studies with radiocontrast have shown leaks often occur through the veins. Other possible routes are through the interosseous circulation, which is not occluded by the tourniquet, and through calcified arteries that the tourniquet fails to occlude.*

The following sentence suggests a lack of ordered thought (and a total ignorance of grammar).

> Of the two amputations which required revision to an above knee level, one was subject to urinary incontinence and trauma in a demented patient, and the other was performed for deep ulceration of the calf muscles.

The word *one* refers to *one of the amputations* (the one affected by urine and trauma). When readers reach the word *other* they expect reference to the other *amputation*. But *other* refers to the other *revision*: the revision, not the amputation, was made necessary because of ulcerated muscles.

Rewritten: *Two amputations required revision to above the knee. One amputation was damaged by the patient, who was demented and also incontinent of urine. The other revision was made necessary by deep ulceration of the calf muscles.*

> The operation may be performed using either the transfrontal or transsphenoidal routes, either of which is usually locally satisfactory, but both have a morbidity and hormonal cure is rare and hypopituitarism frequent.

The relative values of the different segments of the sentence are not well defined. This causes difficulty in the second half of the sentence because having read that '. . . both have a morbidity and hormonal cure' it is then a surprise to readers that *hormonal cure* is the subject of *is*. (*Complications* is here a better word than *morbidity*.)

The sentence needs more positive punctuation. A solution is to split the sentence after the first segment and put a semi-colon after *satisfactory*.

Rewritten: *The operation may be performed transfrontally or transsphenoidally. Although both routes have complications, they are usually locally satisfactory; but hormonal cure is rare and hypopituitarism frequent.*

This is easier to understand at first reading, although it can be improved further by changing the wording and altering the order of the ideas (as is done on p. 187).

Simplicity

Try to keep subjects and their verbs together.

> The survey suggests that attempts to attribute differences in health-related behaviour to ignorance on the part of working class people or to their unwillingness to contemplate lifestyle changes are misplaced.

Attempts is separated from *are misplaced* by complex ideas, whose relevance is not revealed until the end of the sentence. If *misplaced* were *justified,* the implications of the survey would be importantly different, and readers should know this from the beginning of the sentence. Moving *are misplaced* to immediately after *attempts* helps: *The survey suggests that attempts are misplaced that attribute differences. . . .* Readers then know the overall conclusion, but simplifying the construction and separating some of the ideas can improve the example further. Note that some would find *working class people* patronizing.

The working class behave differently towards health. From the survey, this is probably not because of ignorance or because of unwillingness to consider changes of lifestyle.

The plural *behave* is used here because the sense is of individual members not of the class as a whole. Consider *The Health Authority disagree among themselves* and *The Health Authority disagrees with the District General Manager* (see p. 147).

Emphasis and connections

Try to start a sentence with a main clause. Just as with adjectives and adverbs, any subordinate adjectival or adverbial phrases or clauses that follow the main clause must be related unambiguously to the nouns, verbs, phrases or clauses that they qualify.

A common habit of medical writers is to begin a sentence with a past participle, for instance *having.* This can be useful but may lead to grammatical absurdities. Take, for example, the correct but rather ungainly sentence:

The doctor, having admitted the patient, examined the abdomen.

Many writers would start this sentence by describing the order of events:

Having admitted the patient, the doctor examined the abdomen.

This is perfectly good but it is easy to make a classical grammatical error, particularly in the passive voice:

Having admitted the patient, the abdomen was carefully examined.

The participle *having* is now 'dangling': it begins a qualifying phrase that readers expect will qualify the first noun of the main clause *the abdomen* whereas it qualifies the person who did the examining. Obvious here, but it may not be. If not so obvious, dangling participles can cause ambiguity.

Designed with a black strap and yellow case with liquid crystal hands, you will be sure to start a craze this winter. Equally suited for men or women, you can get the watch free with five special bottle caps.

It is the watch, not you, that comes designed with black strap, yellow case, liquid crystal hands, and suitably bisexual.

The construction of *having + past participle* is sometimes useful to describe the order in which things were done (see below), but the construction of starting with subordinate clauses should not be used too often. It postpones the main point of the sentence and separates the main point from the phrases and clauses qualifying it, of which this next is an extreme example:

Because of the possibility of danger to swimmers in the pool by the use of plastic footballs, beachballs and handballs, which can easily dislodge the roof lighting and cause injury, as previously advised, these are not permitted in the swimming pool. Staff are asked to note this and also to ensure that their guests do not bring these items into the pool.

The opening *because of* is qualifying *not permitted*, which is near the end of the first sentence. The example has many other faults and is an extraordinarily clumsy way of saying that *Staff must ensure that neither they nor their guests take plastic footballs, beachballs, or handballs into the swimming pool. As we have pointed out before, these items may dislodge the lighting from the roof on to swimmers.*

Starting the next example with the subordinate clause would have avoided ambiguity:

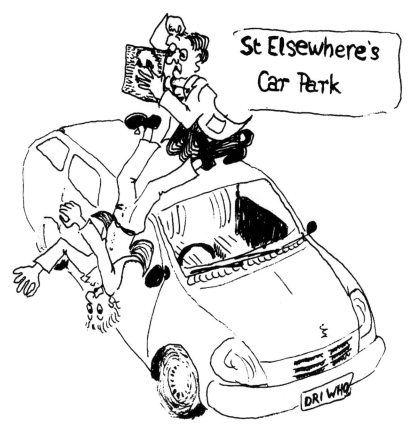

Mr X fell off a car roof because a doctor failed to diagnose a skull fracture.

[The] health authority has been ordered to pay £600 000 damages to [Mr X] who fell off a car roof and suffered severe head injuries because a doctor at [the] hospital failed to diagnose a skull fracture.

Mr X did not fall off the car because of the doctor's failure. A comma before *because* is one solution (and there should also be a comma before *who*), but the subsidiary clause is important. It is better placed at the start of the sentence, and expanded to include the reason for damages: *Because a doctor at [the] hospital failed to diagnose a skull fracture after [Mr X] fell off a car roof and suffered severe head injuries, [the] health authority has been ordered to pay him £600 000 damages.*

> Having established the presence of a pneumothorax and assessed the indications for drainage, the radiological localisation of the air pockets permits the clinician to manoeuvre . . .

The clinician, not the localization of air, assesses the indications for drainage. Use of the passive voice (see p. 139) has caused this inelegant construction. Try: *Once the clinician has established that there is a pneumothorax requiring drainage, better placement is aided by radiological localisation of the air pockets. . . .*

> Except for the oldest and youngest and those with full stomachs, almost all the children were anaesthetised briefly for the caudal injection . . .

It can be helpful to start with an exception if there is only one: *Except for the neonates, all the children. . . .* In the example there are three exceptions, which makes the sentence clumsy. The writer then writes *almost all*, leaving readers wondering whether there were some other exceptions as well. There is more than one way of rewriting this more clearly, but the main idea (that the children were usually anaesthetized) should be presented first. Try: *The children were usually anaesthetised briefly for the caudal injection. The youngest, oldest, and those with full stomachs were usually left awake.*

> Fentanyl 0.1 mg was administered intravenously five minutes before etomidate in order to decrease the pain often found with the injection of etomidate.

Given is better than *administered* (see p. 46) and *in order* is superfluous (see p. 117). The sentence is in the passive voice (see p. 139). Correcting these points is an improvement:

> *We gave fentanyl 0.1 mg intravenously five minutes before etomidate to decrease the pain often found with injection of etomidate.*

This is better but is still clumsy: *etomidate* is written twice (not necessarily incorrect but unnecessary here) and pain is not *found*. The clumsiness is caused partly by this poor choice of words and partly because, contrary to the general rule, the sentence should start with the subordinate idea:

> *To lessen the pain that can occur when etomidate is injected, we gave fentanyl 0.1 mg intravenously five minutes beforehand.*

To return to an example from the section on 'Balance':

The operation may be performed transfrontally or transsphenoidally. Although both routes have complications, they are usually locally satisfactory; but hormonal cure is rare and hypopituitarism frequent.

This is the modification of the original example on p. 182. It can be improved by altering the order of ideas. As it stands, the main idea of the second sentence is the main clause (*they are usually locally satisfactory*), and it has two qualifiers. One is a subordinate clause, a general statement about complications. The other qualifier is two main clauses (*hormonal cure is rare*; *hypopituitarism is frequent*), both of which are important but lose effect tucked away at the end.

The transfrontal and transsphenoidal approaches are usually locally satisfactory, although they are not without complications. However, hormonal cure is rare, and hypopituitarism is frequent.

Sometimes the matter of emphasis between clauses is mostly a matter of punctuation.

There is still argument about the figures, but by any standard contraceptive provision is often inadequate or too expensive.

On first reading, standard is read as qualifying contraceptive, which in turn qualifies provision. The phrase *by any standard contraceptive provision* is read as an aside. Readers then find an unexpected *is* without a subject and have to re-read for the correct sense: a garden path sentence (see p. 166). The basic sense of the sentence is *argument about figures . . . but provision inadequate*. This sense is clear if the comma after *figures* is removed and the true aside *by any standard* enclosed by commas.

Writers should bring out the best in their work, emphasize what they want to be emphasized and connect what they want connected, rather than leave readers to make the emphases and connections. It is hard work and it takes practice to communicate ideas clearly. But if planning a study has taken months and you have spent hours late into the night carrying it out, why not take some trouble in the writing?

The first sentence

The sentence that more than all others needs careful writing is the first sentence of a paper. It is automatically emphasized by its position, and you should think carefully about it. Too many papers start with sentences that can only be described as banal (*COD*: trite, feeble, commonplace); they are the written equivalent of clearing the throat. As the opening sentences of newspaper articles, written for laypeople, these two examples might do well; surely they are not news to their intended readers:

> Despite major advances in the treatment of psychiatric disorders over the last decade outcomes for patients and their families have been found to be less than ideal.

> Virtually all known diseases show variation in rate of occurrence, both temporally and geographically, and it remains a guiding principle of epidemiology that specification of such variation usually provides important clues to the origin and nature of a given disorder.

If diseases did not vary in time and place there would be no such thing as epidemiology.

> The kidneys are bilateral, bean shaped organs, which lie in a retroperitoneal position on either side of the vertebral column beneath the diaphragm.

This sentence is a curious mixture of popular magazine (bean shaped organs, which is better hyphenated: *bean-shaped*) and technical terms (retroperitoneal). It is unnecessary as the opening sentence of a chapter about regional blood flow in a specialized book.

Avoiding abbreviations

A certain way to upset editors, confuse readers and destroy clear prose is to litter your writing with abbreviations. With any abbreviation, one has to ask: what purpose does this serve? Although there are abbreviations that are so well understood that they are almost in themselves part of the vocabulary, in general the only so-called benefit is a spurious saving of space. Abbreviations are useful for chemical names and mathematical terms: DNA, SEM (we mean 'standard error of the mean' not 'scanning electron microscope', which shows that an abbreviation does not mean all things to all people) and so on. They are better if they can be pronounced, in which case they are acronyms; so UNESCO, ANOVA and GABA 'work' better than EDTA and EMG, both of which are often used without explanation in medical papers. But why abbreviate, to give two common examples, haematocrit to Hct and haemoglobin to Hb? Consider the phrase: *A haematocrit of less than 30%. . . .* Is the abbreviation pronounced H . . . c . . . t, or does the reader automatically interpret it as haematocrit? If abbreviated, is it *A Hct . . .* or *An Hct . . .*? Of course it is commonplace, economic and acceptable to use abbreviations for types of haemoglobin (e.g. HbA_2) and abnormal haemoglobins (e.g. HbS, Hb Chad); it is the routine abbreviation of just Hb that is unnecessary. Even with 'accepted' abbreviations, reading is difficult if there are a number in one sentence.

You must also consider readers from outside your own interests, and those whose first language is not English, who may have familiar abbreviations based on words in their language: in French NATO is OTAN, and AIDS is SIDA. Abbreviations and jargon make it more difficult for an 'outsider', and make it easier for 'insiders' to protect themselves. The only purpose of writing is to communicate; if communication is eased by abbreviations, then they are useful. We believe that communication is often clouded by abbreviations.

Of those abbreviations peculiar to medicine, some are accepted by almost everyone, for instance CVP is fairly standard for central venous pressure, but it is still better to use as few abbreviations as possible. All you are doing is saving ink and paper at the cost of ease of comprehension, and you can probably save as much or more by taking care with the writing. In fact, there are five different spelled-out forms for CVP in a well-known book of medical abbreviations. Careful editors will make sure that all but those abbreviations acceptable to the journals are explained at first use. The abbreviations listed in Baron's *Units, Symbols and Abbreviations* (see Reference books, p. 240) are more likely to be widely understood. The list is 'necessarily arbitrary' and should not be seen as giving permission to use an abbreviation. What is important is the context of the abbreviation and the number used.

Established abbreviations (by which we mean either 'standard' or acceptable to a particular editor) can be manipulated like words. So plurals such as PGs (prostaglandins) are feasible if not universally welcomed. Similarly, abbreviations can become possessives (general practitioner's surgery becomes *GP's surgery*). But it is an abuse to make abbreviations into covert strings of modifiers (see p. 163). *COAD patients* is not any better than *chronic obstructive airways disease patients*; possibly it is worse.

Some object to the noun *X-ray* as an abbreviation for radiological examination, and object even more strongly to the verb *to X-ray*, although both the noun and the verb are in the *COD*. Now that radiological examination includes computer tomography and magnetic resonance imaging, X-ray is a reasonable term to use for a standard filmed or screened exposure. However, just as one writes *CT scan* or *MRI scan*, so one should write *X-ray film* for the product of the examination. Radiograph is preferred for X-ray film by many publishers; there is no corresponding verb.

There is seldom a need to use abbreviations, even in abstracts or conference proceedings where there is a limit to the number of words. A passage full of abbreviations is a sign of a lazy or hurried writer, not a marker of good scientific content. Abbreviations make writing cluttered and difficult to understand.

> Laryngoscopy and intubation increased SAP, HR and SVR and decreased SV. Q was unchanged. The increase in HR was greater in N and UT, while the decrease in SV was greater in group N compared with group B. The patients in group B exhibited substantially slower resting HR and a smaller increase to L + I than in group UT.

Readers should not need a glossary to understand your writing, even if, as here, it is 'only' a conference abstract. This preliminary report of scientific work requires as much care as any other scientific writing. In full papers, because the summaries are often the only part of a paper that is actually read (and because summaries are taken verbatim by electronic scientific databases), it is particularly important to explain any abbreviations used in them. Some journals do not allow abbreviations in their summaries.

Readers should not have to remember what group N, group B and group UT are. SVR and SV are poorly chosen abbreviations because SV stands for different words in the two abbreviations. It is the job of a writer to communicate clearly, not in the fewest possible lines. Rewriting this passage in full may lengthen it a little, but makes it understandable even to someone not wishing to read the rest of the abstract.

> *Laryngoscopy and intubation increased blood pressure, heart rate and peripheral resistance but decreased stroke volume. Cardiac output was unchanged. Rate increased most in the normotensive and untreated patients. Stroke volume decreased more in the normotensives than those treated with beta-blockers. The resting heart rates were lower in the treated than untreated patients, and responded less to the stimulus.*

Did the workers who wrote this next sentence take as little care with their science as with their writing?

Bup-induced depression of cardiac contractility and impulse conduction is enhanced in the presence of therapeutic concentrations of Dil.

Rewritten with care but without the idiotic and illiterate abbreviations, the sentence is shorter than the original.

Therapeutic concentrations of diltiazem worsen the depressive effect of bupivacaine on cardiac contractility and conduction.

The ill-chosen acronym in this example appeared in a Lancet editorial: 'Chain of events required for PERVs to pose public-health threat.' It is not easy to see why *pig endoviruses* was not preferred.

Some very common abbreviations of Latin expressions litter medical writing: e.g., *exempli gratia*, for example; etc., *et cetera* (literally 'and the rest'), and so on; i.e., *id est*, that is. There are more elegant alternatives to 'e.g.' and 'i.e.' (see p. 138). The abbreviation 'etc.' can be avoided by using *such as, and so on* or other constructions. A particular abbreviation, not peculiar to medicine but almost universal in medical texts, is *et al.*, which is abbreviated Latin and means *and others*. Some journals proscribe it. We dislike it because, in general, foreign phrases or their abbreviations (particularly the less common ones such as *v. infra, re, ibid.* and *passim*) are better replaced by the English equivalents. *Vide infra* means *see below*; *re* means *about* or *concerning*; *ibid* short for *ibidem* and sometimes shortened further to *ib.*, appears most commonly in reference lists meaning 'in the same work as above' – and is useful used in this way; *passim* appears in text to mean 'and further quotations or reference to the same work' – there is usually a way of expressing this simply, depending on the context, without using *passim. Smith and co-workers* is a reasonable way of avoiding *et al.*

This leads, inter alia, to retinal detachment.

Inter alia means, and is better written, *among other things.*

A digression into other Latin expressions is justified here. A particular horror is to write of patients being examined *on an ad hoc basis*. This is usually written instead of *as necessary, as indicated* or *as convenient*, although *ad hoc* actually means (*COD*): for a particular, usually exclusive, purpose. (See also BASIS.)

Three other Latin expressions that appear in medical English are in vivo, in vitro and *in situ*. (The use of italic or roman style for such terms is usually decided by the publisher.) The first two are excellent ways of expressing succinctly what they mean (taking place in a living organism; taking place in a test-tube or other laboratory equipment) but the third is usually a pompous substitution for *in place*. Some radiotherapists wrote '... the vaginal applicator should be kept *in situ*...' to which one can only reply that a vaginal applicator is not very useful outside you; flippant perhaps, but ill-chosen words often cause unexpected associations – and doctors who treat cancer should be particularly careful not to misuse *in situ* because of its use in the apposite technical term 'carcinoma *in situ*'.

Numbers within text can be given as figures, a form of abbreviation, rather than spelled out, although house style (see p. 12) will dictate what appears in print. You should, however, be consistent in your manuscript. Spell out numbers under ten unless they refer to measured units: so '1 ml' and '5 ml' (no full stops) are correct, but it should be *one patient* and *three days*. Spell out numbers that begin a sentence, writing the units in full: *One millilitre of arterial blood.* . . . With this scheme, starting a sentence *1048 specimens were examined* . . . is incorrect, but spelling out 1048 is cumbersome; such sentences can always be rewritten to avoid the problem: *Altogether, 1048 specimens.* . . . Some journals, including the *Lancet*, seem happy to start sentences with figures.

Ten millilitres as the subject of a verb may take either the singular or plural (see p. 108); *1048 specimens* always takes the plural (unless *A total of 1048 specimens* . . .) (see p. 147).

15
Drawing clear graphs

We have urged that the maxim for good medical writing is the shorter word in the shorter construction. The same applies to illustrations: they should be simple; they should show what you want to show and no more; they should be honest and not distort your results; and they should be clear at first reading. This chapter outlines how to produce the most common type of illustration in medical scientific papers, the diagrammatic representation of numerical data: the graph. There is instruction on other types of illustration in some of the books in the bibliography; and we will not be giving more than the very simplest of statistical advice.

Tufte (see Reference books, p. 240) uses the idea of data-ink and non-data ink: ink that is needed to indicate a number, and ink that is embellishment. In his comprehensive book, *The Visual Display of Quantitative Information*, he writes, 'Just as a good editor of prose ruthlessly prunes out unnecessary words, so a designer of statistical graphics should prune out ink that fails to present fresh data-information.' The main reason for non-data-ink is the increasing use of computer packages, which produce all types of fancy diagram at the tap of a keyboard. A magazine review of an upgraded graphic package began: 'Presentation is about creating an impression, so it is of prime importance to get the material just right.' For many users of these packages – business people in selling and advertising – style is as important, or even more important, than substance. For scientists, the substance is all that matters. If they use graphic packages inappropriately, they do nothing to improve the already poor presentation of much scientific data. Bernard Dixon[39] was writing of slides presented at meetings when he wrote, '[in] a typical, glitzy business presentation . . . the medium truly is the message, as tawdry and vacuous sentiments are given a patina of momentous significance. The average scientific meeting, by comparison, is likely to show at least half a dozen examples of the reverse – lots of content, appalling presentation.'

Scientific numbers are either counted (patients treated, days in hospital, beds occupied) or represent measured variables (blood pressure, cardiac output, serum calcium). With few data in your paper, the best way to show your results may be simply to incorporate the numbers into the text itself. The more data there are, the more useful is a graph. Text consisting of strings of numbers, each with their units, standard deviations and ranges, and each number referring to different subgroups and different variables, is almost impossible to understand at first glance. Sometimes a table is better than a graph. If in doubt, prepare both (not difficult with computer packages) and show them to someone unconnected with the study.

Counts are often single but may be summary (average number of patients treated, days in hospital); measurements are usually summary (blood pressures of a sample of 25 patients, serum calciums of 10 patients before and after taking calcium-lowering drugs). With small samples, the best graphic representation may be to show all the data, each as a discrete point. With larger samples, summary counts or measurements should be represented by an index of the central tendency (for example the median or the mean) and an index of the dispersion around that central tendency (for example the interquartile range or the standard deviation). Sometimes an index of likelihood (for example the 95% confidence limits) is more appropriate than an index of dispersion. These indices are mathematically related, and statistical texts give advice on which to use when.

Counts are best shown by histogram (column graph) and measurements by points (scatter plot or line graph). Measurements are commonly but incorrectly illustrated by column graphs, often because they are the preselected, or 'default', setting of the computer package. Column graphs of measurements can be misleading, especially when the upright axis (y-axis: ordinate) does not go down to zero.

Around each column or point, the dispersion or likelihood is shown as a line (often referred to as an 'error bar', which is a misnomer but a useful generic expression). Every graph must be accompanied by a legend that enables readers to understand the graph without having to search the text, although repetitive statistical detail is best dealt with by a comment to *see text*. The legend must give a succinct summary of what is shown; it must explain all the symbols used and all abbreviations, which in contrast to the text (see p. 188) are often necessary in graphs. If succeeding graphs are

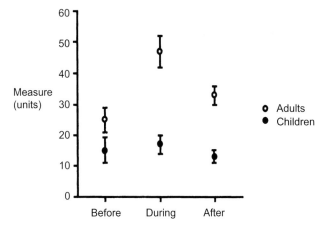

Figure 15.1 Measurement in appropriate units (means and 95% confidence intervals) before, during and after the investigative procedure. Adults (n = 37) are shown as open circles and children (n = 26) as filled circles. Adults' values were consistently higher than children's values, and there were statistical differences between the periods (see text).

similar, some journals allow the comment *for details see Fig . . .*, but others require a full legend for every graph.

Figure 15.1 (note 'Figure' spelled out to start the sentence and the addition of the chapter number if figures are to be numbered by chapter) is a typical simple and clear graph for a measurement that varies over the course of a procedure, and which is different in adults and children. [The legend gives the general idea of how to write a legend, not the specifics of a particular study. Many journals do not require the symbols to be explained on the graph *and* in the legend, and will usually use the actual symbols, not their verbal descriptions, in the legend. Explication of results in the legend is barred by many journals, especially if it repeats the text.]

Next is a typical simple and clear graph (Fig. 15.2) for a count that varies over a period of time, and which is different in adults and children. Note that the legends to Figs. 15.1 and 15.2 contain explicit information (and that house style here puts a full point after Figs.). Patients assigned to study groups are often referred to as, for example, *group A* and *group B* instead of *adults* and *children*. This is not helpful either in the text (see p. 189) or in graphs. The same is true for axis labels: *before, during and after* is better than *I, II and III* or some similar contraction.

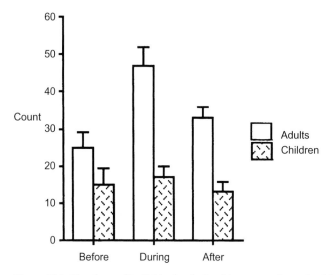

Figure 15.2 Numbers of individuals admitted (means and standard deviations) to 25 hospitals before, during and after a public health action. Adults are shown as clear boxes and children as hatched boxes. Adults were seen consistently more often than children, and there were statistical differences over the period of investigation (see text).

Figure 15.3 illustrates the same numerical data as in Fig. 15.2, but with some faults. Instead of numbers being represented by columns, they are represented by blocks (three-dimensional columns). But the extra dimension, depth, adds no information and with the error bars on top makes the whole thing look like a series of detonation plunger boxes. (Tufte argues that the height of a column is the only necessary information, and that the width of a column is as redundant as the depth. This is true: but the resulting graphs have a skeletal appearance, and do not enable the useful distinction between counts and measurements given by histograms and line graphs when used appropriately.) The top and side surfaces of the blocks have no meaning but are shaded differently from the front surface – which is the only surface that holds information. The shading is poorly chosen: harsh diagonals, especially when juxtaposed, cause neuro-optical swimming sensations. Dotted or dashed patterns (as in Fig. 15.2), or varying shades of grey, are easier on the eye.

There are other distractions. It is best if all writing on a graph is in the same typeface (font), particularly as publishers of journals have largely

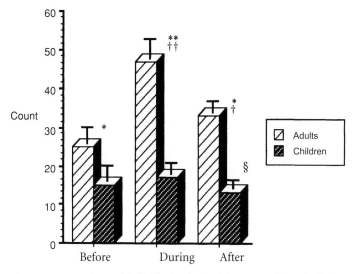

Figure 15.3 Numbers of individuals admitted (means and standard deviations) to 25 hospitals before, during and after a public health action. Adults are shown as light hatching and children as heavy hatching. Adults were seen consistently more often than children (*p < 0.05; **p < 0.01). There were differences within the adults (†p < 0.05; ††p < 0.01) and within the children (§p < 0.05) over the period of investigation.

abandoned the relabelling of submitted artwork to a uniform style and tend to take it straight 'to camera'. Helvetica, used in Figs. 15.1 and 15.2, is often recommended. In Fig. 15.3, the writing is in different fonts (the *y*-axis values are Helvetica). The *x*-axis labels are not aligned. The legend is unnecessarily in a box. The *y*-axis has too many tick marks. The major marks, marking off intervals of 10, are enough; the minor marks, at intervals of 2, do not enable more precision. The numbers should be given explicitly in the text if the numbers need to be known more precisely.

The final potential distraction in Fig. 15.3 is the statistical information, given as symbols *, **, and §. These symbols are helpful if there are few comparisons, but become more confusing the more comparisons there are.

Three-dimensional column graphs are bad enough. Some programs allow the whole graph to be rotated in any of the three dimensions. In Fig. 15.4, meaningless but distorting perspective is added to what should be a simple representation of the number of beds filled by routine cases on

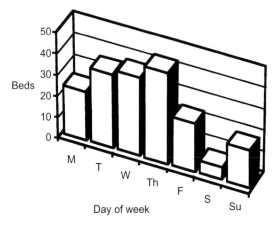

Figure 15.4 Number of beds occupied in the surgical unit by routine cases by day of the week.

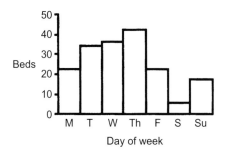

Figure 15.5 Number of beds occupied in the surgical unit by routine cases by day of the week.

the different days of the week. Each column is separated from the next, and each is placed neatly on a surface: neither the separation nor the surface has any meaning. Looking at the graph, you half expect to see people peering around the corner of the 'skyscrapers'; or perhaps it is a cut-away shoebox with children's bricks piled up in it.

Figure 15.5 presents the same information as Fig. 15.4 but with less ink, all of which is data-ink.

Graphs should not contain too much information: six sets of data for one graph is the maximum, and even that may be too much. Figure 15.6 contains four sets of data, each marked by a different symbol – but, contrary to expectations, different types of line do not make interpretation easier. The eye follows the four individual solid lines of Fig. 15.7 more

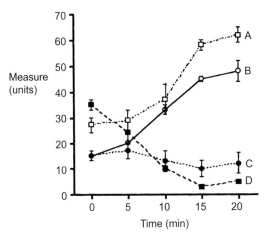

Figure 15.6 Measurements (units) of four biochemical activities after drug was given at time 1 minute. Open squares: A; open circles: B; filled circles: C; filled squares: D. Changes in A, B and D were statistically significant (see text).

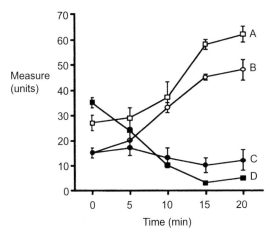

Figure 15.7 Measurements (units) of four biochemical activities after drug was given at time 1 minute. Open squares: A; open circles: B; filled circles: C; filled squares: D. Changes in A, B and D were statistically significant (see text).

easily than the solid, dashed or dotted lines of Fig. 15.6. (Be consistent with symbols between related graphs.)

Illustrations can be almost uninterpretable if the error bars overlap between a number of different lines. It helps to delete either the upper

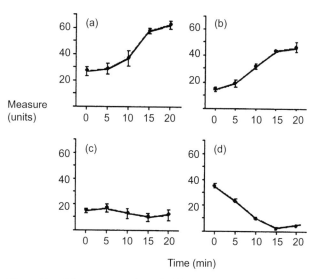

Figure 15.8 Measurements (units) of four biochemical activities after drug was given at time 1 minute. Top left: (a); top right: (b); bottom left: (c); bottom right: (d). Changes in (a), (b) and (d) were statistically significant (see text).

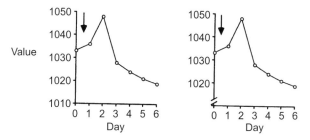

Figure 15.9 The change in the value of a variable over time. The arrow denotes an intervention, which, after a latent period of 2 days, causes the variable to decrease. The position of the curve relative to zero is shown in the right-hand graph by the break in the y-axis.

or lower half of each bar, but if that does not separate the lines clearly enough consider presenting each graph separately in a block of graphs (Fig. 15.8). Remember that the excuse 'error bars have been omitted for clarity' can be interpreted to mean, 'Our results were all over the place'.

It is easy to misrepresent data in graphs, especially by altering the scales on the axes. Most packages will preselect the scale simply from the range of values. In Fig. 15.9, the smallest value is just less than 1020 and the largest

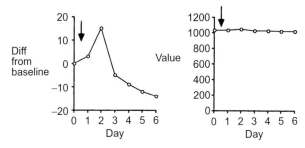

Figure 15.10 The change in the value of a variable over time. The arrow denotes
an intervention, which, after a latent period of 2 days, causes the
variable to decrease. The left-hand graph shows the change from
baseline (day 0); the right-hand graph shows the absolute value,
with zero shown on the *y*-axis.

just less than 1050. The program has preselected a default *y*-axis scale of
1010 to 1050, which makes the absolute size of the change of the value
over days 0 to 6 look larger than it is. This is known as 'suppression of the
zero'. Putting a break in the *y*-axis draws the attention of readers to the real
position of the curve.

Another way to misrepresent data is to plot changes from baseline
instead of absolute values (Fig. 15.10, left). No matter how the *y*-axis is
scaled, there is no getting away from the truth: the value does not change
much (Fig. 15.10, right). This, unfortunately, does not stop some investigators trying to alter readers' perceptions. Ultimately the representation
depends on a clinical, not a mathematical or statistical, decision. If a small
absolute change makes an important clinical difference, or if the value is
tightly controlled within only a small range, then a magnified *y*-axis may
be best.

For further discussion of misrepresentation of data, we refer you to any
good textbook of statistics.

Reprise

Computer programs for statistics and drawing are now extremely versatile.
You can represent your data almost any way you want. Cricket Graph™
(Cricket Software, Inc) is one such package and in their manual they have
an Appendix (A) of ten rules. The appendix is titled 'Do's and don'ts of

creating effective graphs'. Rule number one, because 'software developers [are] stumbling over each other to give the consumer literally hundreds of options while creating graphs', is *Simplify*. After listing the other nine, they say again that rule number one is the one to watch most. **KEEP IT SIMPLE!** The capital letters and the bold typeface are quotations from the manual as much as the words – which we will repeat: keep your graphs simple.

PART III

Practice: recuperation

16
Some examples rewritten

Writing improves with practice.

All the following examples need rewriting. Most contain words or phrases commonly used in poor writing, discussed in earlier sections of this book. We indicate these 'marker' words or phrases, and any style fault if appropriate, after each example. Example 1 is invented, all the others are taken from medical books or journals. Some of the passages have been modified slightly to make them more generally understandable but the modifications have not altered the constructions.

If you wish to test yourself with these examples, without seeing our suggestions for rewriting, then turn to the Appendix, where the examples are reproduced without the rewrites.

Example 1

> In the case of this particular elderly patient hypertensive population, reduction of blood pressure by 18/11 mmHg was achieved for a mean duration of follow up period of 4.4 years. However, with regard to overall mortality, there was no effect nor was there any effect on the incidence of occurrence of myocardial infarction, whether of fatal or non-fatal nature. With respect to cardiovascular accidents, a reduction in incidence of 42% was encountered, and this was mainly associated with strokes leading to fatality or serious neurological sequelae. Although it was not significant, cardiovascular mortality was shown to be reduced by 22%.

Markers: IN THE CASE OF, ACHIEVED, HOWEVER, WITH REGARD TO, NATURE, WITH RESPECT TO, ENCOUNTERED, ASSOCIATED WITH, FATALITY, WAS SHOWN TO BE

Style fault: CIRCUMLOCUTION, PASSIVE, NOUNS AS ADJECTIVES, REPETITION

Comment: Many of the words and phrases are superfluous or are substitutions for simpler words. The worst have been marked.

Rewritten: In these elderly patients with hypertension, blood pressure decreased by 18/11 mmHg for a mean follow up of 4.4 years. There was no effect on overall death rate or on the incidence of fatal or non-fatal heart attacks, but there were 42% fewer strokes, mainly apparent in fatal and major strokes. Deaths from cardiovascular disease decreased by 22%, but this was not statistically significant.

Example 2

> There were 41 hospitalizations, with similar numbers in the three day and five day treatments (18 and 23, respectively).

Markers: HOSPITALIZATIONS, RESPECTIVELY

Comment: Typical ugly and awkward medical prose, which seems somehow to ignore that we are dealing here with people. The *hospitalizations* are patients, who were not in treatments but were in groups receiving either three-day or five-day (hyphens help here) treatment.

Rewritten: Forty-one patients were admitted to hospital, 18 from the three-day treatment group and 23 from the five-day group.

Example 3

> The superiority of 18-gauge catheters has not previously been demonstrated.

Markers: SUPERIOR TO (here as superiority of), DEMONSTRATE

Style fault: PASSIVE

Comment: *Previously* and *previous*, *earlier* (and sometimes *early*) have become coded indicators of judgements on past – usually precedent (*COD*: taken as a guide or justification) – studies in medicoscientific writing (see p. 20). When accompanied by a reference they are sometimes ambiguous and often unnecessary; a reference must by implication be to a study that predates the present one. When used to hint that the 'previous' study was a poor one they are wholly unacceptable.

Rewritten (depending on the sense): It is not known if 18-gauge catheters are better.

This is the first time 18-gauge catheters have been shown as better.

Example 4

The new scan typically detects more fractures, plain films detect more malalignments; the two modalities performing in a complimentary fashion.

Markers: MODALITIES, PERFORMING
Style faults: POOR WORD CHOICE, BALANCE
Comment: Use the poor choice of word as a marker: is there a way of restructuring the sentence so *modalities* and *performing* are not needed? There are three segments, but the separating punctuation is incorrect. Semi-colons separate segments of equal value that could themselves be sentences, but the segment that follows the semi-colon could not be a sentence. Complimentary should be complementary; misalignments is better than malalignments.
Rewritten: It is worth using both scans because the new scan is better for diagnosing fractures and plain films for diagnosing misalignments.

Example 5

Until recently, no scientific methodology has been available to assess symptoms or objective degree of genitourinary prolapse; without such methodology the design of clinical trials has been problematic.

Marker: METHODOLOGY
Style faults: WORD CHOICE, REPETITION, BALANCE
Comment: The semi-colon is correct: it separates two segments of equal value that could themselves be sentences but which are too closely connected to have a full stop between them. However, the semi-colon is unnecessary because the example can be rewritten. The problem is the order of thoughts: the first clause is the explanation for the second, and turning the example around makes things neater.
Rewritten: Clinical trials have been difficult to design because there is no method for assessing the symptoms or objective degree of genitourinary prolapse.

Example 6

These trials have led to the evidence-based introduction of several new drugs, some of which have been shown to impact on overall survival.

Markers: IMPACT, SHOWN TO
Style fault: SUPERFLUOUS WORDS
  Comment: We presume, but are not told, whether the impact was good or bad; replacing *to impact on* with *affect* is no better. *Overall* adds nothing to *survival* and *have been shown to* is unnecessary.
Rewritten: These trials have led to the evidence-based introduction of several new drugs, some of which improve survival.
  We wonder what happened to the evidence-based new drugs that have been introduced despite not improving survival.

Example 7

The time-consuming aspects of data collection were minimised by the number of auditors and inconsistencies in coding minimised by the presence of a consultant.

Markers: MINIMIZED, PRESENCE OF
Style faults: PASSIVE, CONNECTIONS
  Comment: Confusing. The two statements are *time was reduced by having enough auditors* and *inconsistencies were reduced by a consultant*. The way the sentence is written suggests from first reading that *time was reduced by auditors and inconsistencies*. These two ideas need separating. The writers were trying to make the point that inconsistencies were reduced by *one particular* consultant, but the by-phrase passive is an awkward way of expressing this.
Rewritten: Having enough auditors reduced the time spent collecting the data. One consultant supervised the coding to try to prevent inconsistencies.

Example 8

Once a fistula has been identified there are several methods employed to localize it; all of which are invasive.

Marker: EMPLOY(ED)
Style faults: TENSES, POOR WORD CHOICE, PUNCTUATION
Comment: The shorter the form of the verb the easier the reading, with less likelihood of grammatical error. It may not be appropriate here, but when giving instruction *Once a fistula is* . . . is more direct than *Once a fistula has been. . . . Ways* is arguably a better and certainly a shorter word than *methods* here. The semi-colon should be a comma, separating the main clause from the relative clause that follows (see p. 177).
Rewritten: Once a fistula is identified there are several ways to localize it, all invasive.

Example 9

Differential rates of gastric emptying of solid and liquid phases have been demonstrated.

Marker: None.
Style fault: PASSIVE
Comment: The need to express difference, with words such as *various, variable* (and VARIABILITY, see p. 93), *different* and *differential*, arises often and can be a problem. *Different* is subtly different from *differential* (*COD*: varying according to circumstances, constituting a specific difference, relating to specific differences (as in differential diagnosis)), and none of its meanings was intended here. *Phases*, a precise meaning in physical chemistry, is unnecessary.
Rewritten: Solids and liquids leave the stomach at different rates.

Example 10

The extent of the differentials in wealth and health, however, can be shown to vary both temporally and geographically, indicating that a reduction in these inequalities is achievable.

Marker: HOWEVER, ACHIEV(ABLE)
Style fault: SUPERFLUOUS WORDS, PASSIVE
Comment: Tim Albert, who runs courses on communication (and see Reference books, p. 240), describes his 'pub test'. Writers of this type of prose are asked what they would say to a drinking companion, sitting in

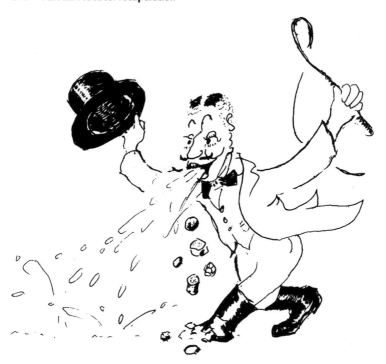

Differential rates of gastric emptying of solids and liquids have been demonstrated.

the lounge bar. This statement could provoke only, 'Eh?' Differential is used here correctly (see above).

Rewritten: Differentials in wealth and health have varied over the years and between different countries, which shows that inequalities can be reduced.

Example 11

Cells were challenged with potassium in the absence or presence of test drugs.

Marker: ABSENCE OF, PRESENCE OF

Comment: Writing *in the absence/presence of* is a common inflation; substituting with/without is nearly always satisfactory, although we, in common with some editors and publishers, dislike the slash mark, most common in *and/or* (see p. 178).

Rewritten: Cells were challenged with potassium, with and without test drugs.

This is not quite correct, because it fails to stress the important experimental point that the test drugs were added before the potassium challenge.

Rewritten: Cells, exposed or not to the test drugs, were then challenged with potassium.

Example 12

Before basing any conclusions on such information it has been necessary to validate measurements with respect to repeatability and reproducibility of its determination.

Marker: SUCH, WITH RESPECT TO

Style fault: CIRCUMLOCUTION

Comment: This sentence is full of the sort of phrases that are unfailing indicators of inflated style: an unnecessary qualifying clause (*before basing*), an inappropriate passive (*it has been necessary*), *with respect to*, and big words with little meaning (*validate, repeatability, reproducibility, determination*). When writing of measurements, repeatability and reproducibility are the same. The writers should have been more explicit if they wished to distinguish repeatability, in the sense of how practical it is to repeat the test, from whether repeat testing gives the same result.

Rewritten: Any conclusions depend on the accuracy of the measurement.

But perhaps this is a statement of the obvious, explaining the obfuscatory style of the original.

Example 13

The health authority has been ordered to pay £600 000 damages to Mr X who fell off a car roof and suffered severe head injuries because a doctor at the hospital failed to diagnose a skull fracture.

Marker: None.

Style fault: WORD ORDER

Comment: Presumably, given a correct diagnosis, the man would not have climbed onto the car roof in the first place. This is a simple grammatical error, caused by the misassociation of *because* with *suffered* rather than with *ordered*. It is the same sort of error as the hanging participle (see p. 185).

Rewritten (1):   The health authority has been ordered to pay £600 000 damages to Mr X because a doctor at the hospital failed to diagnose a skull fracture after Mr X fell off a car roof and suffered severe head injuries.

Mr X has to be repeated, because otherwise the mistake recurs, it seeming that the doctor fell off the car. An alternative is to reverse the sentence, putting the subsidiary clause first.

Rewritten (2):   Because a doctor at the hospital failed to diagnose a skull fracture, the health authority has been ordered to pay . . .

Example 14

The function of the teeth is essentially to facilitate and optimize the eating process.

Markers: FUNCTION, ESSENTIALLY, PROCESS
Style faults: POOR WORD CHOICE, CIRCUMLOCUTION
Comment: A statement of the even more obvious than example 12. Sometimes the obvious does need stating, but this opening sentence of the Introduction to a paper should have been removed as 'throat clearing' (see p. 187). We have reworked it to show that a short, sharp sentence is more effective than cloaking the statement in spurious polysyllables.
Rewritten (1,2,3):
Eating is easier if you have teeth.
Teeth make it easier to eat.
Teeth aid eating.

Example 15

At the aetiological level, an obvious link between dystonia and psychosis exists in the putative role of dopaminergic mechanisms in both.

Markers: AETIOLOG(ICAL), EXISTS, ROLE
Style fault: SUPERFLUOUS WORDS
Comment: Can a putative (*COD*: reputed, supposed) role be an obvious link?
Rewritten: Dystonia and psychosis may both have a dopaminergic mechanism.

Example 16

Certain surgical procedures are known to be capable of inducing malignant tumours, although the ways in which this can happen have been classified as rare and very rare.

Marker: KNOWN TO BE
Style faults: SUPERFLUOUS WORDS, WORD CHOICE, PASSIVE
Comment: *Are known to be capable of* means *can.*
Rewritten: Certain surgical procedures can induce malignant tumours, although rarely.

Classification of the different ways in which surgery causes tumours should follow in another sentence.

Example 17

Release was measured in 6–8 day retinoic acid 10 mM differentiated, monolayer cultured cells.

Marker: None
Style faults: NOUNS AS ADJECTIVES
Comment: This thick stack of modifiers is regrettably not an extreme example of inappropriate striving for economy of words without concern for meaning.
Rewritten: We measured release in a monolayer of differentiated cultured cells incubated for 6–8 days in 10 mM retinoic acid.

If this is not what the investigators meant, they have only themselves to blame.

Example 18

Untreated hypertension especially with an associated tachycardia will detract from this method of management for cardiac patients.

Marker: None
Style faults: CIRCUMLOCUTION
Comment: There is incorrect use of an unfamiliar word: *detract* (*COD*): take away from a whole, reduce credit due to, depreciate. The parenthesis needs separating from the main idea by punctuation. *Associated* is used correctly.

Rewritten: Untreated hypertension, especially if there is an associated tachycardia, makes this method of management less suitable.

Less formally, *especially with tachycardia* will do.

Example 19

> . . . with efficient monitoring of trials and continuous improvements of viral vectors, gene therapy may still represent an important addition to the treatment armamentarium for a range of diseases. . . .

Marker: REPRESENT, ARMAMENTARIUM
Style faults: WORD CHOICE
Comment: The order of thoughts seems back to front: surely the viral vectors should be improved before the clinical trials? A *range of diseases* means no more than *many diseases*. Continual (repeated) is better than continuous (without a break).
Rewritten: . . . with continual improvements of viral vectors and efficient monitoring of trials, gene therapy may still provide useful treatments.

Example 20

> There can be little doubt that the mortality rate of hospital inpatients is increased as a result of urinary tract infections associated with the use of indwelling urinary catheters.

Marker: MORTALITY, AS A RESULT OF, ASSOCIATED WITH, THE USE OF
Style faults: WORD CHOICE, SUPERFLUOUS WORDS
Comment: *Mortality* is sometimes correct, so is *mortality rate*, but not here. *There can be little doubt* can be an appropriate introduction, but always ask of this type of wording: 'Does it add anything to the simple statement?'
Rewritten: Patients are more likely to die in hospital if they contract an infection because of an indwelling urinary catheter.

Indwelling is necessary, to distinguish from single-episode or intermittent catheterization.

Example 21

> . . . all patients with chronic heart failure should be monitored on a regular basis – at least every six months in the case of stable patients.

Marker: BASIS, IN THE CASE OF
Comment: Two of the commonest symptoms of poor medical writing.
Rewritten: . . . all patients with chronic heart failure should be followed up regularly – at least six monthly for patients who are stable.

Patients should have regular follow-up (the hyphen is not essential) avoids the passive. The dash should be used with care but is correct here.

Example 22

Pleural air is commonly missed and even when noted its volume is misleadingly underestimated.

Marker: NOTED
Style faults: SUPERFLUOUS WORDS
Comment: *Noted* is often superfluous (in phrases such as *It was noted that . . .*, see p. 77); here it means *seen* or *noticed*. *Misleadingly* is unnecessary – the volume is bound to mislead if underestimated.
Rewritten: Pleural air is commonly missed and even when noticed the volume tends to be underestimated.

The sense remains if the sentence is shortened: *Pleural air is commonly missed or the volume underestimated.*

Example 23

No currently available methodology exists to monitor continuously the status of regional myocardial revascularization in the postoperative patient.

Marker: METHODOLOGY, MONITOR, EXISTS
Style faults: CIRCUMLOCUTION, SUPERFLUOUS WORDS
Comment: *In the postoperative patient* is *postoperatively, No currently available methodology* is *no current method* or even *no way,* but *It is not yet possible* is better still.
Rewritten (1):   It is not yet possible to continuously measure regional revascularization of the myocardium postoperatively.

Yes: we are splitting an infinitive (see p. 167). We find the alternative awkward: *It is not yet possible to monitor regional revascularization of the myocardium continuously postoperatively.* But if a sentence is awkward, it is a clue that its construction is poor. *It is not yet possible to . . . measure* can be rephrased *Measurement is not yet possible. . . .* The awkward adverbs *continuously* and *postoperatively* can now be shortened.

Rewritten (2): Continuous postoperative measurement of regional myocardial revascularization is not yet possible.

Example 24

> The purpose of this investigation was to determine which of a person's projected palm or whole hand area is a better approximation to 1% of their total body surface area.

Marker: DETERMINE

Style faults: WORD CHOICE, SUPERFLUOUS WORDS

Comment: *To determine an approximation* is *to estimate.* To make it more direct, remove the impersonal *purpose of this investigation.*

Rewritten: We wanted to know whether the palm or the whole hand was the best estimate of 1% of total body area.

Example 25

> The effectiveness of mammographic screening for breast cancer depends on its ability to detect and to exclude the presence of breast cancer, measured as the sensitivity and specificity of mammography, respectively.

Marker: PRESENCE OF, RESPECTIVELY

Style faults: WORD CHOICE, SUPERFLUOUS WORDS, TAUTOLOGY, REPETITION

Comment: There is no need to repeat mammography. Sensitivity and specificity are not the easiest measures to understand, so it is unwise to separate them from their everyday synonyms.

Rewritten: The effectiveness of mammography depends on how well it detects cancer (its sensitivity) and how well it excludes cancer (its specificity).

Better to repeat *cancer* than to have another *it* in the sentence.

Example 26

> Their use saves nursing time in clinic and would reduce the additional cost involved if district nurses are required to remove the sutures as an outpatient.

Marker: INVOLVED
Style faults: CONNECTIONS, SUPERFLUOUS WORDS
Comment: *Their use* is no better than *they*. *Involved* is superfluous. There is a false connection: *district nurses . . . as an outpatient*: the patients, not the district nurses, are outpatients. There is jumbling of singulars and plurals (district nurses, outpatient) and of tenses (saves, reduce).
Rewritten: They save nurses' time in clinics, and save the cost of employing district nurses to remove sutures.

Example 27

The advantages of epidural opiates for the relief of postoperative pain have been repeatedly emphasised. There remains, however, considerable uncertainty as to the consistency and quality of analgesia provided by this technique.

Marker: HOWEVER, AS TO
Style faults: CIRCUMLOCUTION, REPETITION
Comment: *. . . have been emphasised repeatedly* is better than *. . . have been repeatedly emphasised*, but *. . . are well known* is better still. The phrase *by this technique* is unnecessary. *Considerable uncertainty* is *less certainty*.
Rewritten: The advantages of epidural opiates for the relief of postoperative pain are well known although the consistency and quality of analgesia are less certain.

Example 28

At the junction of sutures and staples, however, a meaningful comparison was thereby available. Further, by randomisation of the distribution, a more extensile appraisal of the scar segments could be made.

Marker: HOWEVER, MEANINGFUL, THEREBY
Style faults: SUPERFLUOUS WORDS, CIRCUMLOCUTION, CONNECTIONS, PASSIVE
Comment: Choice of words is poor: *appraisal* should be *assessment*; *extensile* means *capable of being extended*, like a spring or rubber band. The writers presumably thought extensile an impressive way of writing extensive – though even extensive is wrong. *Better* is the needed word,

because randomisation of sutures and staples increased the scientific validity of the study. It is written in the passive voice. *Meaningful* is meaningless.

This example needs rewriting completely. First, delete or alter the poor words.

Rewritten (1):   At the junction of sutures and staples, a comparison was available. Further, by randomisation of the distribution, a better comparison of the scar segments could be made.

Now alter the passive to the active; find better wording for *At the junction of . . .*; and improve the connection between *distribution* and what is being distributed.

Rewritten (2):   We could compare sutures and staples where they were next to one another, and increased the validity of the comparison by randomising their distribution.

Example 29

> Medical directors of NHS trusts may recognise that they have skill deficits, but although these may be addressed when someone is in post, a proactive approach would undoubtedly be preferable.

Marker: ADDRESSED

Comment: Apart from *addressed* (and perhaps *preferable* used instead of *better*), there is nothing that we can put our finger on, but the sentiment can certainly be better expressed. Note the managerial buzzword *proactive*.

Rewritten: It is better for medical directors of NHS trusts to make sure they have all the necessary skills before they take up their posts.

Example 30

> This case can serve as paradigmatic of the working party's approach. Thus, the perspective adopted involves considering the issues with a cost-and-benefits approach in mind.

Marker: PARADIGM

Style faults: CIRCUMLOCUTION, NOUNS AS ADJECTIVES

Comment: A fusion of managementspeak and medicalese, heralded by the inappropriate *paradigm(atic)* and fulfilling its promise with the turgid *perspective adopted* and the awkward *cost-and-benefits approach*.

Rewritten: This case is typical of the working party's approach, which is to consider the balance between cost and benefits.

Example 31

A recent report described the development and implementation of procedures for the management of extravasation of antineoplastic agents resulting in the prompt and uniform treatment of such events.

Marker: SUCH
Style faults: SUPERFLUOUS WORDS, CIRCUMLOCUTION
Comment: At least the writer did not write of *procedure development and implementation* or *antineoplastic agent extravasation management.* Nash[40] commented: 'I ask my doctor to cure me or help me get better, not to provide me with help and guidance concerning the recuperative process.'
Rewritten: The development of how to deal with extravasation of agents used in the treatment of cancer, including a standard scheme for prompt treatment, was described in a recent report.

Note that we prefer the passive *The development . . . was described* to the active *The report . . . described.* This is an example of the doer of an action being unimportant (see p. 139).

Example 32

The sample of 101 women contained three elements. First, the majority (64) typically remanded for reports after conviction. The second element was a small number of women who were charged with arson. . . . Finally, there were the disturbed young women, remanded for minor offences. . . .

Marker: CONTAINED, ELEMENTS, MAJORITY
Style faults: BALANCE
Comment: This exercise is a list (see p. 175) that is in the correct order but incorrectly balanced. There are three items, each item being a number of women. An *element* is irreducible and clearly defined, and not a good word to apply to a number: *group* is better. However, the sample did not *contain* three groups; the groups were *defined later* within the sample. The three items are not (grammatically) balanced: the second two are sentences, but the first item lacks a finite verb (*remanded* is an adjectival participle). The two sentences are not balanced either, because one has a

singular subject and verb (*element was*) and the other the plural (*were*). *The majority* (see p. 73) here is over 51. *More than half* is better.

Rewritten: There were three groups identified in the sample of 101 women. The first, containing more than half the women (64), had typically been remanded for reports after conviction. The second was a small number of women charged with arson. . . . Finally, there was a group of disturbed young women, remanded for minor offences. . . .

> *Example 33*
>
> It could be that the patients already had good oesophageal speech, they were medically unfit or were thought to be too old to cope with the voice prosthesis or simply that by now, they had learned to cope with their communication disability.

Marker: None

Style faults: BALANCE, CONNECTIONS

Comment: This is also a list. The items are *speech, medically unfit, too old* and *learned to cope*. Punctuation must separate the items: as it stands, there are not enough commas and the second comma comes incorrectly within the last item. The first *that* can govern all four items. *Patients* can act as a single subject for which all the items are adjectival clauses; there is no need for subsequent pronouns.

Rewritten (1):   It could be that the patients already had good oesophageal speech, were medically unfit, were thought too old to cope with the voice prosthesis, or had simply learned to cope with their communication disability.

This gives four items that are grammatically equal segments (see p. 179), but there are other ways of writing this, which give different emphases.

Rewritten (2):   It could be that the patients already had good oesophageal speech, were medically unfit or thought too old to cope with the voice prosthesis, or that they had simply learned to cope with their communication disability.

Now medical fitness and age are not separate items but are linked items in causing failure to accept the prosthesis. Repeating the subject (*patients*, as the pronoun *they*) puts extra stress on the last item. Note that repeating the subject demands repetition also of *that*, to maintain grammatical equivalence.

Example 34

Both the techniques of abdominal closure, and the materials to be used, continue to excite debate. Like many others we employ interrupted mass closure, but the best suture method is debatable. Materials such as polyglycolic acid may be associated with a higher rate of late wound failure than non-absorbable materials such as nylon, but the latter may cause wound pain and sinuses.

Marker: EMPLOY, ASSOCIATED WITH, LATTER
Style faults: CONNECTIONS, SUPERFLUOUS WORDS
Comment: Repetitive and wordy, for instance *continue to excite debate.* There is an ambiguous connection: is it both *(the two) techniques of abdominal closure,* or both *the techniques and the materials,* that are under consideration? The writers then write of *the best suture method,* but their next sentence makes it apparent that they meant *suture material.* In *wound failure* and *wound pain* the noun *wound* is used unnecessarily as an adjective. It is better to write of the *formation of sinuses.* Note that *such* is used correctly (see p. 137).
Rewritten: There is still debate about the technique of abdominal closure and about the material to use. We use interrupted mass closure, as do many others, but there is uncertainty about the best suture material. Late failure of wounds is more likely with materials such as polyglycolic acid, but non-absorbable materials such as nylon may cause pain and the formation of sinuses.

Example 35

The detector comprises an oscillating crystal coated with a layer of silicon oil, whose oscillation frequency alters as a result of increases in the mass of the layer in the presence of vapour. The change in oscillator frequency is proportional to the vapour concentration. By the use of an electronic system consisting of two oscillator circuits, one of which has an uncoated (reference) crystal and the other a coated (detector) crystal, an electronic signal can be obtained which is proportional to the vapour concentration.

Marker: COMPRISES (although correct), AS A RESULT OF, PRESENCE OF, USE OF
Style faults: CIRCUMLOCUTION, REPETITION

Comment: Too long (84 words) and repetitive. Cutting this passage down to size means first working out the flow of ideas: a crystal – silicon oil – frequency altered by vapour –two circuits – proportional signal. This, and the next exercise, are not easy to rewrite simply by cutting out a word here and there; they are hard work.

Rewritten: The detector is an oscillating crystal coated with a layer of silicon oil. Vapour, by changing the mass of this layer, alters the frequency of oscillation proportionally to the concentration of the vapour. The proportional electronic signal is obtained by using two oscillator circuits, one having an uncoated (reference) crystal and the other a coated (detector) crystal.

[57 words: from 84]

Example 36

It may have been inferred from the figure on page 226, that at high flows the flow control knob would become unduly sensitive – a small increase in flow producing a disproportionate rise in inflation pressure.

Fortunately, however, the flow rate control has an alinear response, the control becoming less sensitive at high flows. As a result, a conveniently linear relationship is established between the amount of rotation of the flow control knob and the inflation pressure which is produced.

Marker: HOWEVER

Style faults: CIRCUMLOCUTION, NOUNS AS ADJECTIVES, REPETITION, SUPERFLUOUS WORDS

Comment: This passage is verbose [76 words] mainly because of repetition of the same ideas in different words; for example, if the control is unduly sensitive then a small increase in flow must produce a large rise in pressure. In *flow control knob* (see Nouns as adjectives, p. 162), *regulator* may be better than *control* and *knob* is unnecessary. The phrase *inflation pressure* also contains a noun used as an adjective but it seems as useful as *blood pressure* or *prescription charge*. (Some people maintain that *high flows* should be *high rates of flow*. Flow is measured as unit volume per unit time so *rate* is unnecessary; we do not write *rates of speed*.)

Rewritten: Although the figure on page 226 shows that at high flows a small increase in flow produces a disproportionate rise in inflation pressure, the flow control is alinear, so there is a linear relationship between rotation of the control and the inflation pressure.

[40 words]

This can be reduced further to:

At high flows, a small increase in flow produces a disproportionate rise in inflation pressure (see figure on page 226) but, because the flow control is alinear, the relation between rotation of the control and inflation pressure is linear.

[36 words]

Example 37

> In summary, foam filled endotracheal cuffs would appear to offer a preferable alternative to low pressure high volume cuffs in terms of protecting the airway and this efficacy is achieved in the context of cuff to tracheal wall pressures that are both predictable and acceptable.

Marker: IN TERMS OF, ACHIEVED

Style faults: CIRCUMLOCUTION

Comment: An excellent example of using more and longer words than necessary: *in the context of* means *with*; *would appear to offer a preferable alternative* means *are better than*. There are long strings of modifiers: *foam filled endotracheal cuffs*, *low pressure high volume cuffs*, and *cuff to tracheal wall pressures*. In general, if modifiers of this form are used, we prefer them hyphenated, e.g., low-pressure high-volume.

Rewritten: In summary, foam-filled endotracheal cuffs protect the airway better than cuffs with low pressure and high volume. The pressure between the foam-filled cuff and the tracheal wall is predictable and acceptable.

Example 38

> It is possible to speculate that operative intervention would have saved this man's life. The policy of management was conservative because of uncertainty as to the cause of the deterioration.

Marker: None

Style faults: CIRCUMLOCUTION, REPETITION

Comment: At first sight this looks like a bureaucratic inflation of medical writing. But we suspect that medicolegal considerations led to obscurity as a strategy to avoid blame, a strategy becoming more common in medical texts (see p. 20). Note the three levels of hedging: *possible* . . . *speculate* . . . *would.* The repetition is in stating that management was conservative when this is implicit in the first sentence.

Rewritten: An operation might have saved this man's life, but we did not operate because we did not know why he had deteriorated.

Example 39

> The inequalities in the provision of medical care cannot be defended in terms of provision being demand determined, since the ability of patients to express needs as demands is conditional upon the availability of services.

Marker: IN TERMS OF

Style faults: NOUNS AS ADJECTIVES, CIRCUMLOCUTION

Comment: A sentence should be clear on first reading. On first reading, the initial suggestion is that inequalities may depend on an aspect of demand being determined *by something*. It takes some time to realize that *provision being demand determined* does not mean *demand determined by something*, but *provision being determined by demand*. Using the noun *demand* as an adjective is confusing.

One thing can be *described* in terms of another but it cannot be *defended* in terms of something.

The physicist Richard Feynman was a clear thinker who used clear language. He quoted a sociologist who wrote 'The individual member of the social community often receives his information via visual, symbolic channels,'[8] which, as Feynman pointed out, means *people read*: an example of saying a lot and meaning not much. The example above comes from writers interested in 'health resources'; their motives may be more sinister. Were the writers trying to conceal that they had nothing to say? Or, were they trying to prevent readers from understanding the true meaning, like the militarists who referred to civilians killed by 'incontinent ordnance'?[12] (See euphemism and p. 16).

Rewritten: The inequalities in the availability of medical care are not simply because of inequalities in demand, because patients cannot demand what is not available.

Readers may have their own ideas of what the original means.

Example 40

Each case has to be managed individually after a full history has been taken, and examination and, where necessary, special investigations have been undertaken, so that an accurate diagnosis can be made and appropriate treatment selected.

Style faults: SUPERFLUOUS WORDS, PASSIVE, PUNCTUATION
Comment: The commas are scattered at random. Read this aloud and the inappropriate pauses are obvious. There are superfluous words.
Rewritten: Each case has to be managed individually. A full history and examination and any necessary special investigations will enable an accurate diagnosis and appropriate treatment.

Example 41

Baby walkers are devices that provide preambulatory infants with postural support in addition to offering them the opportunity to experience bipedal locomotion. They are intended to simulate independent walking and by so doing, it is argued, encourage and even accelerate the early acquisition of this skill.

Marker: None
Style faults: CIRCUMLOCUTION
Comment: Why call a spade a spade when it is so easy to call it a two-handed long-handled digging implement? And yet there are no markers within the passage, and a grammar checker passed it.
Rewritten: Baby walkers are devices that allow babies who are still at the crawling stage to stand and to practise walking. Some authorities believe that they speed up the ability of babies to walk independently.

Example 42

The doctor's life is the life of a person. One would expect medical education to assume this truth as self-evident and give the doctor preparation not only by providing an optimum environment for gaining knowledge and skill but also by encouraging personal growth.

Marker: ENVIRONMENT
Style faults: WORD CHOICE, CLICHÉ

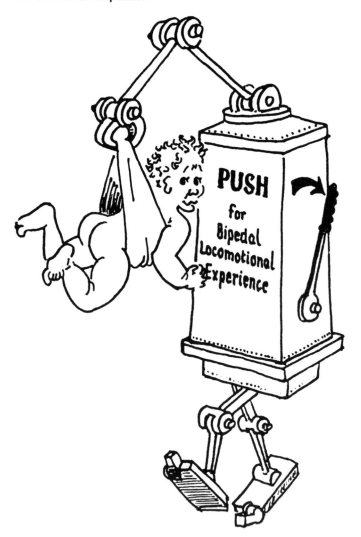

. . . opportunity to experience bipedal locomotion.

Comment: These are the opening sentences of a 'mission statement' for a medical school. Does anyone take this sort of stuff seriously, other than the people who write it? The sentiment is laudable, but for some reason it is felt that writing it in ordinary words means it will not be taken seriously. **Rewritten:**   Doctors are people too. A medical education is not just about the best way of learning knowledge and skills, but about how to cope with all the things that life throws at you.

Yes, this is informal and almost chatty – but it's better than personal growth. If you were a prospective medical student, which would appeal to you more?

Example 43

Theories of cognitive psychology addressing fundamental limitations of cognition offer an explanation for the occurrence of this phenomenon in terms of attentional resource allocation. For example, fundamental cognitive principles indicate that unless a heavily-loaded clinician in the operating theatre specifically allocates attentional resource to the perception of (say) the oxygen saturation numeric, the only thing that the clinician will be able to reliably report about the numeric is its colour.

Comment: We offer this as a last example, without guidelines to its dissection and reconstruction. Either the reader will by now have some idea that this all-too-typical style is inflated and an obstacle to communication, or we have failed. We notice that our deflation gives a more realistic view of the clinician – a movement from the rhetoric of infallibility of the original to a more humane and accessible alternative.

Rewritten: Because of the way the human brain works, if clinicians in the operating theatre have a lot to think about then, unless they make a conscious effort to take note of the oxygen saturation, all that registers is the colour of the display.

Postscript to the examples

It is a sad reflection on the process of education that medical graduates – after 13 years at school, 5 years at university, and perhaps 10 or more years as postgraduates – express themselves in the way they do. What possesses medical writers that they have to write *bipedal locomotion* instead of *walking*?

An anonymous assessor of the first edition of this book wrote, 'They are never taught to write. Multiple choice questions have a lot to answer for. They do not have time to read well.' Doctors should make time to read well; there is more to life than medicine.

No one should attempt a project in medical research without taking time to read published work or to learn the required techniques; everyone expects that the analysis will require a knowledge of the appropriate statistics; yet ultimately the message depends on the writing. It makes sense to take as much care with the writing as with any other aspect of research. For review articles it is even more important that the writing is clear.

17

Do the experts agree?

Experts in the use of English argue about details as much as experts in medical subjects argue about the details of physiology, diseases and treatments. While in the preparation, parts of the first edition of this book were seen by many people. Changes made after the suggestions of one expert were often criticized by another. Books about English usage offer differing advice.

Look up the use of hyphens: 'There are clear rules about the use of a hyphen' and 'There are no hard and fast rules . . .'.

The use of *as* or *since* to mean *because* is, according to one authority, 'not acceptable'. According to another, '*as* is perfectly good English; but should be replaced by *while* or *because* if there is the possibility of confusion'. This last quotation has a semi-colon followed by *but*, yet there is advice that a semi-colon should never be followed by *but*.

'Never start a sentence with *however*' from one authority can be countered by another who holds that 'Some pedantic users of English object to the use of *but* and *however* as the first word of a sentence' and dismisses the argument for this as having 'little to recommend it'.

Some object to *X-ray* and *biopsy* as verbs. The *COD* has them as verbs.

There are differences of opinion even on spelling. One book has '-ize should be preferred to -ise when both endings are in use' and another has 'acceptance of -ise is now general, and is recommended as a means of avoiding error'.

Some consultant editors object strongly to any use of nouns as adjectives, but action potential, road traffic accident, blood supply, and plasma sodium are all neat and sensible. Invoking absolute grammatical rules to condemn this use of nouns is unhelpful. Helpful advice is suggesting that it is not overdone, because it can be clumsy and ambiguous: when the headline in a local newspaper read 'Babies in food scare' it did not mean that babies had been discovered in food.

These are details. All experts – whatever their opinions about hyphens, *since, however, to biopsy,* or *plasma sodium* – would criticize the authors who wrote:

> Such events [air emboli] are everpresent realities in a busy clinical environment where the various plastic components of necessity are manipulated and disconnected by a variety of the nursing staff.

What are *plastic components of necessity?*

In plain English, and there is no reason to write anything else, the example means *This* [air embolus] *is always possible on a busy ward where nurses of varying experience have to manage intravenous equipment.*

To quote from Phythian: 'Ultimately it is usage that determines the nature of English. Usage may be criticised, condemned and resisted; but in the last resort, dictionaries and grammar books have to record what is, not what ought to be. What is standard practice in a language is governed by what is habitual, i.e. by usage.'

Language is not an inanimate, unchanging, thing. But we shall be sad if future medical editors and medical audiences require writers and speakers to cloak their meaning in polysyllabic fog – referring to wards as clinical environments, to likelihoods as everpresent realities – and prefer this 'pseudodignified prose'[17] to clarity.

Appendix: examples to rewrite

Example 1

In the case of this particular elderly patient hypertensive population, reduction of blood pressure by 18/11 mmHg was achieved for a mean duration of follow up period of 4.4 years. However, with regard to overall mortality, there was no effect nor was there any effect on the incidence of occurrence of myocardial infarction, whether of fatal or non-fatal nature. With respect to cardiovascular accidents, a reduction in incidence of 42% was encountered, and this was mainly associated with strokes leading to fatality or serious neurological sequelae. Although it was not significant, cardiovascular mortality was shown to be reduced by 22%.

Example 2

There were 41 hospitalizations, with similar numbers in the three day and five day treatments (18 and 23, respectively).

Example 3

The superiority of 18-gauge catheters has not previously been demonstrated.

Example 4

The new scan typically detects more fractures, plain films detect more malalignments; the two modalities performing in a complimentary fashion.

Example 5

Until recently, no scientific methodology has been available to assess symptoms or objective degree of genitourinary prolapse; without such methodology the design of clinical trials has been problematic.

Example 6

These trials have led to the evidence-based introduction of several new drugs, some of which have been shown to impact on overall survival.

Example 7

The time-consuming aspects of data collection were minimised by the number of auditors and inconsistencies in coding minimised by the presence of a consultant.

Example 8

Once a fistula has been identified there are several methods employed to localize it; all of which are invasive.

Example 9

Differential rates of gastric emptying of solid and liquid phases have been demonstrated.

Example 10

The extent of the differentials in wealth and health, however, can be shown to vary both temporally and geographically, indicating that a reduction in these inequalities is achievable.

Example 11

Cells were challenged with potassium in the absence or presence of test drugs.

Example 12

Before basing any conclusions on such information it has been necessary to validate measurements with respect to repeatability and reproducibility of its determination.

Example 13

The health authority has been ordered to pay £600 000 damages to Mr X who fell off a car roof and suffered severe head injuries because a doctor at the hospital failed to diagnose a skull fracture.

Example 14

The function of the teeth is essentially to facilitate and optimize the eating process.

Example 15

At the aetiological level, an obvious link between dystonia and psychosis exists in the putative role of dopaminergic mechanisms in both.

Example 16

Certain surgical procedures are known to be capable of inducing malignant tumours, although the ways in which this can happen have been classified as rare and very rare.

Example 17

Release was measured in 6–8 day retinoic acid 10 mM differentiated, monolayer cultured cells.

Example 18

Untreated hypertension especially with an associated tachycardia will detract from this method of management for cardiac patients.

Example 19

. . . with efficient monitoring of trials and continuous improvements of viral vectors, gene therapy may still represent an important addition to the treatment armamentarium for a range of diseases. . . .

Example 20

There can be little doubt that the mortality rate of hospital inpatients is increased as a result of urinary tract infections associated with the use of indwelling urinary catheters.

Example 21

. . . all patients with chronic heart failure should be monitored on a regular basis – at least every six months in the case of stable patients.

Example 22

Pleural air is commonly missed and even when noted its volume is misleadingly underestimated.

Example 23

No currently available methodology exists to monitor continuously the status of regional myocardial revascularization in the postoperative patient.

Example 24

The purpose of this investigation was to determine which of a person's projected palm or whole hand area is a better approximation to 1% of their total body surface area.

Example 25

The effectiveness of mammographic screening for breast cancer depends on its ability to detect and to exclude the presence of breast cancer, measured as the sensitivity and specificity of mammography, respectively.

Example 26

Their use saves nursing time in clinic and would reduce the additional cost involved if district nurses are required to remove the sutures as an outpatient.

Example 27

The advantages of epidural opiates for the relief of postoperative pain have been repeatedly emphasised. There remains, however, considerable uncertainty as to the consistency and quality of analgesia provided by this technique.

Example 28

At the junction of sutures and staples, however, a meaningful comparison was thereby available. Further, by randomisation of the distribution, a more extensile appraisal of the scar segments could be made.

Example 29

Medical directors of NHS trusts may recognise that they have skill deficits, but although these may be addressed when someone is in post, a proactive approach would undoubtedly be preferable.

Example 30

This case can serve as paradigmatic of the working party's approach. Thus, the perspective adopted involves considering the issues with a cost-and-benefits approach in mind.

Example 31

A recent report described the development and implementation of procedures for the management of extravasation of antineoplastic agents resulting in the prompt and uniform treatment of such events.

Example 32

The sample of 101 women contained three elements. First, the majority (64) typically remanded for reports after conviction. The second element was a small number of women who were charged with arson. . . . Finally, there were the disturbed young women, remanded for minor offences. . . .

Example 33

It could be that the patients already had good oesophageal speech, they were medically unfit or were thought to be too old to cope with the voice prosthesis or simply that by now, they had learned to cope with their communication disability.

Example 34

Both the techniques of abdominal closure, and the materials to be used, continue to excite debate. Like many others we employ interrupted mass closure, but the best suture method is debatable. Materials such as polyglycolic acid may be associated with a higher rate of late wound failure than non-absorbable materials such as nylon, but the latter may cause wound pain and sinuses.

Example 35

The detector comprises an oscillating crystal coated with a layer of silicon oil, whose oscillation frequency alters as a result of increases in the mass of the layer in the presence of vapour. The change in oscillator frequency is proportional to the vapour concentration. By the use of an electronic system consisting of two oscillator circuits, one of which has an uncoated (reference) crystal and the other a coated (detector) crystal, an electronic signal can be obtained which is proportional to the vapour concentration.

Example 36

It may have been inferred from figure 2 that at high flows the flow control knob would become unduly sensitive – a small increase in flow producing a disproportionate rise in inflation pressure. Fortunately, however, the flow rate control has an alinear response, the control becoming less sensitive at high flows. As a result, a conveniently linear relationship is established between the amount of rotation of the flow control knob and the inflation pressure which is produced.

Example 37

In summary, foam filled endotracheal cuffs would appear to offer a preferable alternative to low pressure high volume cuffs in terms of protecting the airway and this efficacy is achieved in the context of cuff to tracheal wall pressures that are both predictable and acceptable.

Example 38

It is possible to speculate that operative intervention would have saved this man's life. The policy of management was conservative because of uncertainty as to the cause of the deterioration.

Example 39

The inequalities in the provision of medical care cannot be defended in terms of provision being demand determined, since the ability of patients to express needs as demands is conditional upon the availability of services.

Example 40

Each case has to be managed individually after a full history has been taken, and examination and, where necessary, special investigations have been undertaken, so that an accurate diagnosis can be made and appropriate treatment selected.

Example 41

Baby walkers are devices that provide preambulatory infants with postural support in addition to offering them the opportunity to experience bipedal locomotion. They are intended to simulate independent walking and by so doing, it is argued, encourage and even accelerate the early acquisition of this skill.

Example 42

The doctor's life is the life of a person. One would expect medical education to assume this truth as self-evident and give the doctor preparation not only by providing an optimum environment for gaining knowledge and skill but also by encouraging personal growth.

Example 43

Theories of cognitive psychology addressing fundamental limitations of cognition offer an explanation for the occurrence of this phenomenon in terms of attentional resource allocation. For example, fundamental cognitive principles indicate that unless a heavily-loaded clinician in the operating theatre specifically allocates attentional resource to the perception of (say) the oxygen saturation numeric, the only thing that the clinician will be able to reliably report about the numeric is its colour.

References and further reading

References

1 Furedi, F. *Where Have all the Intellectuals Gone?* London: Continuum, 2004, p. 95.

2 Dixon, B. (ed.) *From Creation to Chaos: Classic Writings in Science.* Oxford: Blackwell, 1989.

3 Anonymous. Superstring theory. *Lancet* 1989; ii: 426–7.

4 Durant, J. Silver tongues and twitching eyebrows. *The Times Higher Educational Supplement* 25 Mar 1994, pp. 21–2.

5 Shuster, S. Loneliness of a long distanced reviewer. *Br. Med. J.* 1981; 283: 1443–4.

6 Perutz, M. *Is Science Necessary? Essays on Science and Scientists.* London: Barrie and Jenkins, 1989.

7 Medawar, P. *Memoir of a Thinking Radish.* Oxford: Oxford University Press, 1986.

8 Feynman, R. P. *'Surely You're joking, Mr Feynman!'* London: Unwin, 1986.

9 Gregory, M. W. The infectiousness of pompous prose. *Nature* 1992; 360: 11–2.

10 O'Donnell, M. One man's burden. *Br. Med. J.* 1985; 290: 250.

11 Barrass, R. *Scientists Must Write.* London: Chapman & Hall, 1978.

12 Lutz, W. The world of doublespeak. In Ricks, C., Michaels, L. (eds.) *The State of the Language,* 1990 edition. London: Faber and Faber, 1990.

13 Dutton, D. B. *Worse Than the Disease: Pitfalls of Medical Progress.* Cambridge: Cambridge University Press, 1988.

14 Silverman, W. A. *Human Experimentation: A Guided Step into the Unknown.* Oxford: Oxford University Press, 1985.

15 Anonymous. Surrogate measures in clinical trials. *Lancet* 1990; 335: 261–2.

16 Whimster, W. F. Reading, writing – and rewriting. *Br. Med. J.* 1987; 294: 1011.

17 Anonymous. Trimming hedges. *Lancet* 1992; 340: 275–6.

18 Tinker, J. H. Book review. *N. Engl. J. Med.* 1994; 330: 946.

19 Hayes, D. P. The growing inaccessibility of science. *Nature* 1992; 356: 739–40.

20 Pickering, G. *High Blood Pressure,* 2nd edn. London: Churchill, 1968.

21 Watson, J. D., Crick, F. H. C. A structure for deoxyribose nucleic acid. *Nature (Lond)* 1953; 171: 737–8.

22 Whimster, W. F. Be your own subeditor. In *How to do it: 1*, 2nd edn. London: BMJ Publishing Group, 1985, pp. 220–3.

23 *MacUser* 9 July 1993, p. 55.

24 Anonymous. Personal view: a hidden handicap. *Br. Med. J.* 1994; 308: 66–7.

25 Bloom, D. A., Mory, R. N., Hinman, F. Jr. Dilation vs. dilatation. *J. Urol.* 1992; 147: 1682

26 Aronson, J. K. "Where name and image meet" – the argument for adrenaline. *Br. Med. J.* 2000; 320: 506–9.

27 Crick, F. *What Mad Pursuit: A Personal View of Scientific Discovery.* London: Weidenfeld & Nicolson, 1988.

28 Mitchell, J. R. A. Back to the future: so what will fibrinolytic therapy offer your patients with myocardial infarction? *Br. Med. J.* 1986; 292: 973–8.

29 Paton, A. Way with words. *Br. Med. J.* 1994; 309: 253.

30 Brewin, T. B. Empirical: one word, two meanings. *J. R. Coll. Phys. Lond.* 1994; 28: 78–9.

31 Burkhart, S. Sexism in medical writing. *Br. Med. J.* 1987; 295: 1585.

32 Kuhn, T. *The Structure of Scientific Revolutions*, 2nd edn. Chicago: University of Chicago Press, 1970.

33 Goodman, N. W. Paradigm, parameter, paralysis of mind. *Br. Med. J.* 1993; 307: 1627–9.

34 Up & down the city road. *The Independent Magazine*, 5 Feb 1994, p. 10, col 3.

35 Eger II, E. I. A template for writing a scientific paper. *Anesth. Analg.* 1989; 68: 740–3.

36 Ziman, J. *Reliable Knowledge.* Cambridge: Cambridge University Press, 1978, p. 42.

37 Howard, P. *Winged Words.* London: Corgi, 1983.

38 Pinker, S. *The Language Instinct.* London: Allen Lane, Penguin Press, 1994, pp. 213–14.

39 Dixon B. Slide rules. *Br. Med. J.* 1994; 309: 1665.

40 Nash, W. *English Usage. A Guide to First Principles.* London: Routledge and Kegan Paul, 1986.

Reference books

Everyone needs a dictionary. The bookshops are not short of them. Each to their own, but we recommend the one that we have generally referred to in the text, the *COD*, of which the latest edition is:

Soanes, C., Stevenson, A. (eds.) *Concise Oxford English Dictionary*, 11th edn. Oxford: Clarendon, 2004.

Also necessary is:

Baron, D. N. (ed.) *Units, Symbols and Abbreviations. A Guide for Biological and Medical Editors and Authors*, 5th edn. London: Royal Society of Medicine Services, 1994.

There are two general style books revered for their time in print: *Plain Words* first appeared in 1954, 'to help officials in their use of written English'. They still need help. The first incarnation of Strunk and White is even earlier: it was published in the USA in 1918.

Gowers, E. *The Complete Plain Words.* 3rd edn, revised by Greenbaum, S., Whitcut, J. London: HMSO, 1986.

Strunk, W. I., White, E. B. *The Elements of Style.* Harlow: Longman, 1999.

These are some short general books, whose titles are self-explanatory:

Bryson, Bill. *Troublesome Words.* Harmondsworth: Penguin, 2002.

Hicks, W. *Quite Literally. Problem Words and How to Use Them.* New York: Routledge, 2004.

Trask, R. L. *Mind the gaffe. The Penguin Guide to Common Errors in English.* London: Penguin, 2002.

Trask, R. L. *The Penguin Guide to Punctuation.* London: Penguin, 2004.

There are books that give advice to writers in science and medicine:

Albert, T. *Winning the Publications Game: How to Write a Scientific Paper Without Neglecting your Patients*, 2nd edn. Oxford: Radcliffe Medical Press, 2000.

> *The author of this book runs courses for health professionals, and his website (http://www.timalbert.co.uk/) is worth a visit.*

Barrass, R. *Scientists Must Write*, 2nd edn. London: Routledge, 2002.

Huth, E. *Writing and Publishing in Medicine*, 3rd edn. Baltimore: Lippincott, Williams & Wilkins, 1998.

O'Connor, M. *Writing Successfully in Science.* London: Routledge, 1991.

Doctors may not write well, but they don't usually write about *kicking into touch* or *hitting the ground running*. Unless they become managers, when they should read this:

Carr, S. *Tackling NHS Jargon. Getting The Message Across.* Oxford: Radcliffe Medical Press, 2001.

Aiming more at those who develop an interest in language, there are larger, more comprehensive reference works.

Burchfield, R. W., Fowler, H. W. *Fowler's Modern English Usage*, revised edn. Oxford: Oxford University Press, 2005.

Weiner, E. S. C., Delahunty, A. *The Oxford Guide to English Usage*, 2nd edn. Oxford: Oxford University Press, 1994.

Dictionaries and style guides are all very well, but they are not good for telling which is correct of large, big and great, or small, little and tiny. Invaluable for that, and especially for non-native speakers is:

Hayakawa, S. I., Ehrlich, E. *The Penguin Guide to Synonyms and Related Words*, 2nd edn. London: Penguin, 1996.

If you want good, clear graphs, this simple book expands the advice given in our chapter:
Bigwood, S., Spore, M. *Presenting Numbers, Tables, and Charts*. Oxford: Oxford University Press, 2003.

For an idea of what it is really possible to do with graphs and charts:
Tufte, E. R. *The Visual Display of Quantitative Information*. Surrey: Graphics Press, 2001.

Books to read or dip into

Language is wonderful. Those who know this already will probably have seen the following books; those who don't know will be convinced by them. They are explanatory and exploratory; you don't have to read them, but they will make you a better person, whether or not your papers get published.

Asher, R., Holland, R. (eds.) *A Sense of Asher*. London: BMJ Books, 1984.

> *Richard Asher was one of the best and most sensible medical writers. This is not a book about how to write; it is a book that shows you how to write.*

Bryson, B. *Mother Tongue. The English Language*. Harmondsworth: Penguin, 1991.

> *The story of the language, told with humour.*

Burchfield, R., Simpson, J. *The English Language*. Oxford: Oxford University Press, 2002.

> *More scholarly than Bryson.*

Crystal, D. *The Cambridge Encyclopedia of the English Language*, 2nd edn. Cambridge: Cambridge University Press, 2003.

> *What it says: encyclopaedic. Read about Singapore English, the great vowel shift and more.*

Crystal, D. *Rediscover Grammar*, 3rd edn. Harlow: Pearson Longman, 2004. A pocket sized, travel guide to grammar.

Honey, J. *Language is Power. The Story of Standard English and its Enemies*. London: Faber and Faber, 1997.

> *A political tract which asks, why, if 'standard English' is decried by so many as elitist, those who support standard English are so keen that everyone should learn it.*

McArthur, T. *Oxford Guide to World English*. Oxford: Oxford University Press, 2003.

> *Covers much of the same ground as the Crystal book (above) but in a more conventional format.*

O'Donnell, M. *A Sceptic's Medical Dictionary*. London: BMJ Publishing Group, 1997.

> *The inventor of the term Decorated Municipal Gothic.*

Pinker, S. *The Language Instinct. The New Science of Language and Mind.* London: Penguin, 1995.

Language, neurophysiology and psychology: a best seller.

Quiller-Couch, A. *On the Art of Writing.* Cambridge: Cambridge University Press, 1916.

(Out of print) This was a standard in its time. Current scholars are prone to complain that it is time we put Quiller-Couch away, but his chapter, 'On the capital difficulty of prose', given to me (NWG) by my D. Phil. supervisor, Bob Torrance, helped to set me on my way to better writing.

Truss, L. *Eats, Shoots and Leaves. The Zero Tolerance Approach to Punctuation.* London: Profile Books, 2003.

Pinker (above) was a best-seller; Truss was, and still is, a phenomenon.

Index

Words or phrases in small capitals in the index are those whose use in medical writing is discussed specifically in the text. Page numbers in **bold** indicate where in the text the main discussion takes place.